Lúcia Maria Torres dos Santos Gil
Isabel Maria Ribeiro Fernandes

Quality of Life for People with Inflammatory Bowel Disease

Lúcia Maria Torres dos Santos Gil
Isabel Maria Ribeiro Fernandes

Quality of Life for People with Inflammatory Bowel Disease

Determining Factors

Imprint

Any brand names and product names mentioned in this book are subject to trademark, brand or patent protection and are trademarks or registered trademarks of their respective holders. The use of brand names, product names, common names, trade names, product descriptions etc. even without a particular marking in this work is in no way to be construed to mean that such names may be regarded as unrestricted in respect of trademark and brand protection legislation and could thus be used by anyone.

Cover image: www.ingimage.com

This book is a translation from the original published under ISBN 978-613-9-75093-1.

Publisher:
Sciencia Scripts
is a trademark of
Dodo Books Indian Ocean Ltd. and OmniScriptum S.R.L publishing group

120 High Road, East Finchley, London, N2 9ED, United Kingdom
Str. Armeneasca 28/1, office 1, Chisinau MD-2012, Republic of Moldova, Europe
Printed at: see last page
ISBN: 978-620-6-42190-0

ACKNOWLEDGEMENT

To my supervisor Professor Isabel Maria Ribeiro Fernandes for her patience, guidance and encouragement in preparing this work.

To my husband and children, for their unconditional love and tolerance of my impatience and absences. For encouraging me and giving me the courage not to give up. For the understanding and patience with which they accompanied me on this journey.

Thank you to my parents for always making me believe that I could do it, for loving and accepting me unconditionally. Thank you for the effort and hard work you put in so that I could realise my dream of becoming a nurse and investing in an area of specialisation.

To my brothers for being my "safe harbour". To my nephews who I love and the rest of my family. Thank you all for your support.

To the people with inflammatory bowel disease who participated willingly, because it was thanks to them that this work was possible.

To all the professors who shared their knowledge and made this master's degree possible.

To my friends and colleagues for their friendship, encouragement and help in times of difficulty and doubt.

To all those who didn't believe it was possible, because they made me stronger and more determined.

To God, my spiritual strength.

I would like to thank all the people and organisations who, directly or indirectly, supported me and allowed this study to come to fruition.

Sincerely, well done to everyone.

SUMMARY

Background: Inflammatory bowel disease usually affects young adults and has a chronic, relapsing clinical course with an impact on quality of life, particularly in aspects related to health, education, work, social and family life. It is one of the main areas of intervention in Gastroenterology. It is globally considered to be a disabling disease and responsible for a marked reduction in the person's quality of life, be it Ulcerative Colitis, Crohn's Disease or Undetermined Inflammatory Disease.

Objectives: To assess the perceived quality of life of people with inflammatory bowel disease, registered at the Outpatient Clinic of a Local Health Unit in the Central Region, and to analyse the determinants of this quality of life.

Methods: This was a descriptive-correlational, cross-sectional, quantitative study aimed at people with inflammatory bowel disease who attended the Outpatient Clinic of a Local Health Unit in the Centre Region. The study sample was consecutive and by convenience, made up of 38 participants. A questionnaire was applied consisting of sociodemographic, clinical and behavioural variables and the Inflammatory Bowel Disease Questionnaire (IBDQ-R) assessment tool, made up of 32 questions that assess four dimensions of quality of life, namely: Intestinal Symptoms; Systemic Symptoms; Emotional Aspects and Social Aspects (Veríssimo, 2008).

Results: The study sample consisted of 19 men and 19 women, with an average age of 43.20 years and with a level of education greater than or equal to the 12th year of schooling (57.80%). In terms of pathologies, they had Crohn's Disease (50.00%), Ulcerative Colitis (26.30%) and Undetermined Inflammatory Bowel Disease (23.70%). The majority were married (65.80%) and were active in the labour market (57.80%). As far as inferential statistics are concerned, it can be concluded that there is a statistically significant relationship between quality of life in the "Social Aspects" dimension and level of education; the existence of hospitalisations and smoking habits, with the latter variable also showing a significant relationship in terms of the values presented in the total IBDQ-R.

This study concluded that people with inflammatory bowel disease have reasonable levels of perceived quality of life, with an average for the total IBDQ-R of 45.80 per cent.

Keywords: Inflammatory Bowel Disease; Quality of Life; Determining Factors.

TABLE OF CONTENTS:

INTRODUCTION

In the field of health, the diagnosis and experience of an illness can give rise to a set of symptoms in people and their families and trigger another level of needs that need to be met. When it comes to chronic illness, feelings of incapacity and difficulty in adapting to new conditions emerge, inherent in the requirement for a significant change in their lives.

Despite the technological advances witnessed in recent years in an attempt to reduce the incidence rates of some chronic diseases, there has been a significant increase with direct and indirect implications for the quality of life (QoL) of those affected and their families. In this sense, nurses are involved in the dynamisation of innovative activities, seeking to provide creative solutions for dealing with situations of chronic illness, aiming to improve the care provided and the need to reduce the associated costs, providing a real difference in the day-to-day life of the person, family and community (Ordem dos Enfermeiros, 2010a).

Inflammatory bowel disease (IBD) is a chronic disease characterised by chronic intestinal inflammation and is subdivided into two main forms, namely Crohn's Disease (CD) and Ulcerative Colitis (UC). CD is a discontinuous, transmural inflammation that can affect any part of the gastrointestinal tract. UC is the most common form and, unlike CD, is restricted to the intestinal mucosa, so it is less susceptible to complications and many patients have a mild disease course (Smeltzer, Bare, Hinkle and Cheever, 2011).

IBD is manifested by intestinal, extraintestinal and systemic symptoms, requiring numerous hospitalisations, admissions and prolonged treatments, which has direct implications for people's well-being, affecting various areas of life, namely physical, psychological and social (Magalhães, Castro, Carvalho, et al., 2015).

Although the aetiology is not entirely clear, according to scientific studies, IBD develops in genetically susceptible people due to the action of environmental factors, which condition a maladjusted and exaggerated inflammatory response to antigens by the immune system (Nunes, Fiorino, Danese and Sans, 2011).

Its incidence and prevalence has increased significantly in different regions of the world, which demonstrates its emergence as a global disease, requiring specific investment in terms of research studies that contribute to the early identification of risk factors and enable specific preventive action (Molodecky, Soon, Rabi et al., 2012).

At European level, the incidence and prevalence of IBD has increased, with the current estimate being approximately 0.30 per cent of the affected population, with a wide geographical variation (Burisch, Jess, Martinato and Lakato, 2013).

This pathology occurs all over the world, representing a serious public health problem and affecting young people from different socio-economic classes, genders and nationalities, who frequently relapse and have highly severe clinical forms, creating major repercussions for people's QoL.

In Portugal, the prevalence of this pathology has been increasing progressively, affecting around 56/100,000 inhabitants (Administração Central do Sistema de Saúde, 2009). According to the National Hospital Speciality and Referral Network (2016), there are some more recent studies that estimate the prevalence of IBD in Portugal to be 150/100,000 inhabitants, with a tendency to increase progressively. This progressive increase in the incidence and prevalence of the disease will have direct consequences for people's well-being and QoL.

The concept of QoL is characterised by subjectivity, which involves the entire human condition, be it physical, psychological, social, cultural or spiritual. This holistic conception of man is the basic foundation for quality nursing care, enabling comprehensive attention to a human being who is more fragile and in need of support and help in meeting their needs, whether in the community or hospital context (Martins, França and Kimura, 1996).

With real knowledge of the implication of a chronic illness on a person's wellbeing and perception of their QoL, this subject is of particular interest for the development of research studies with the aim of obtaining results that will enable changes in individual behaviour and at the level of health professionals.

In this context, the purpose of this research project is to discuss the problems faced by people with "inflammatory bowel disease", in which the aim is to assess their perception of quality of life, seeking to obtain data and make positive contributions to the enrichment and development of nursing.

It is essential to know how to minimise the discomfort and complications of this pathology and enable the large number of people with IBD to have the best possible QoL, avoiding absenteeism from work and consecutive hospitalisations.

The fundamental starting point for any research is to choose an area of interest and transpose it into a question that can be studied, in this case, "What is the Perception of the Quality of Life of People with Inflammatory Bowel Disease", followed in the Outpatient Clinic of a Local Health Unit in the Centre Region. To this end, the following objectives were formulated:

- ✓ To assess the perception that people with inflammatory bowel disease have of their quality of life;
- ✓ To analyse the factors that determine the quality of life of people with inflammatory bowel disease;

In view of the problem under study, we decided to carry out a study that falls within the quantitative research paradigm and is descriptive-correlational, cross-sectional and quantitative.

In this context, the population selected was people with IBD attending the Outpatient Clinic of a Local Health Unit in the Centre Region. The study sample was obtained consecutively and for convenience, taking into account the time frame established for data collection.

This study used a self-administered questionnaire comprising a set of questions including sociodemographic, behavioural and clinical variables, together with a measuring instrument validated for the Portuguese population by Veríssimo (2008), called the *Inflammatory Bowel Disease Questionnaire* (IBDQ-R), revised version, which includes a set of 32 items to assess different aspects of the QoL of people with IBD, grouped into four dimensions:

> Intestinal symptoms;
> Systemic symptoms;
> Emotional aspects;
> Social aspects.

In order to situate the problem in question and frame it methodologically, this dissertation is organised into two main and distinct, but interconnected, parts.

The first part of the study consists of the theoretical background, where the first chapter develops the theme of the disease, with some considerations about chronic disease and IBD, in terms of pathological and epidemiological characterisation. The second chapter conceptualises quality of life, health-related quality of life and the quality of life of people with chronic inflammatory bowel disease, highlighting the role of the Community Nurse Specialist in promoting the QoL of these people.

The second part of the study refers to the development of the empirical study. The third chapter discusses the research methodology used to carry out this study and all its components, namely: the research question, the type of study and its objectives, the research hypotheses, the target population/sample and sampling criteria, the operationalisation of the variables, the data collection instrument and the ethical and data collection procedures. The fourth chapter presents and analyses the results obtained. The fifth chapter discusses the results and finally presents the conclusion and some considerations on the limitations of the study and suggestions for future work, taking into account the data obtained.

Finally, the bibliographical references that served as the basis for this work will be presented.

CHAPTER 1
THEORETICAL BACKGROUND

1 - THE CHRONICALLY ILL PERSON

The appearance of a chronic illness in a person's life implies a process of adaptation to a life characterised by certain constraints, particularly at sentimental, emotional, behavioural and social levels, which translate into family, work and even financial changes. This set of changes has a major impact on the person and their family, requiring the development of specific strategies to facilitate adaptation to the illness process.

The World Health Organisation (WHO) describes "chronic disease as a disease of prolonged duration and slow progression" and describes "chronic conditions as health problems that require continued treatment over a period of years or decades" (OE, 2010a, p.8). It is essential that health professionals understand the seriousness of the problem in order to ensure effective action to promote health, prevent illness and provide appropriate care for patients (OE, 2010a).

According to the Order of Nurses (2010a), these are the health professionals who are best able to help people and their families find creative and transformative solutions to the challenge of chronic illnesses, making a difference in their daily lives; in the process of empowering people to accept their health condition and in developing strategies that facilitate this process, providing a better QoL.

Throughout this process, the support of the family and health professionals, particularly nurses specialising in community nursing, is essential in accepting the chronic illness, encouraging the person to believe in their potential and abilities to cope with the situation, providing them with tools that make it easier to live with and accept the chronic illness. In this sense, the family should play an active role in the care and treatment of their relative, accompanying and supporting them in moments of discouragement, which are very common in these processes.

Chronic illness is seen around the world, and particularly in Europe, as responsible for a large proportion of mortality and morbidity rates, and is expected to increase in the coming years. It often leads to recurrent episodes of hospitalisation due to worsening and decompensation of the disease and/or its consequences/complications. Inadequate management of the disease and the therapeutic regime are the most frequent causes of decompensation, leading to a high number of hospitalisations, which reflects the shortcomings felt in healthcare in order to reduce or even avoid these situations and all the economic and social costs involved, in addition to the losses felt in terms of QoL (Bastos, 2013).

Nurses play an important role in health promotion and disease prevention, contributing to the fight against chronic illness and the process of caring for the millions of people affected worldwide (OE, 2010a).

7

With the development of new technical, scientific and pharmacological technologies, people with chronic illnesses are faced with an increase in average life expectancy, albeit coupled with the experience of a specific symptomatological picture and the appearance of some complications that can have a significant influence on the level of QoL, affecting the individual person and their family (Castro, Ponciano and Pinto, 2010).

Chronic illnesses also affect young people, a reality that is often overlooked by society, which tends to see them as inherent to the elderly. It is a long-term illness, with a very limited chance of cure, in which the person needs to create strategies to adapt to their new living conditions. The impact of the disease on the lives of young adults is more significant than on middle-aged or elderly people. Thus, young people who are at the peak of their productivity are faced with a set of limitations and difficulties that are unusual or not expected at that age, such as the need to see the doctor very often, to comply with a prolonged and continuous therapeutic regime and to be exposed to the risk of suffering from worsening pathologies that require frequent hospitalisations. This condition generates feelings of sadness, anger or apathy, among other symptoms, implying considerable physical and emotional suffering and with implications for their personal, family and social well-being (Castro, et al., 2010).

In adolescence, chronic illness is even more worrying, since young people have specific characteristics and this phase is experienced in a very particular way and often proves to be quite problematic. The relationship that is established between health professionals and these people requires the former to develop communication and relational skills that transcend the needs exclusively related to the experience of the disease process, focusing on the prevention of risk behaviours (Santos, Santos, Ferrão, and Figueiredo, 2011).

It is known, however, that changing lifestyle habits and adopting healthy behaviours early on has great potential for promoting health and minimising the onset of chronic diseases and their complications, and it is important to stop smoking and drinking (Castro, et al., 2010).

Accompanying these people, specifically in the outpatient setting, is a concern for health professionals insofar as the disabilities resulting from the treatments and the wear and tear/suffering of the person and family are easily recognisable and identifiable, together with the frustration felt at the lack of investment in disease prevention and health promotion to the detriment of cure and rehabilitation (Marcon, Radovanovic, Waidman, Oliveira and Sales, 2005).

People with chronic illnesses are confronted immediately after their diagnosis with the need to change some of their lifestyle habits, in particular their adherence to the therapeutic regime, since this is a chronic condition that requires them to take medication for the rest of their lives. In addition to this definitive change in their lives, they also have to learn to deal with the physical, social and family discomfort associated with chronic illness, requiring a process of mutual adaptation on the part of the person and their family, in the search for stability and, consequently, acceptance of the illness (Molodecky and Kaplan, 2010).

Experiencing a chronic illness requires a lot of investment on the part of the person to transform an unpleasant situation into one that implies a new life condition, and it is useful to adopt resilience strategies that provide a healthy, quality way of life, despite all the inherent constraints (Marques, 2012).

Chronic illness is reflected in people's lives in various areas, and its impact on QoL is notorious and significant. There are numerous chronic diseases that affect different systems and organs, and IBD is one of them that is constantly on the rise, hence the interest in studying this subject, which is developed below.

1.1 - INFLAMMATORY BOWEL DISEASE

IBD represents a group of idiopathic chronic inflammatory intestinal disorders that result from the constant and inadequate activation of the mucosal immune system (Torres, Santana, Torres, Moura and Neto, 2011). It takes on the character of an autoimmune disease in its various manifestations, as the immune system itself attacks the body's healthy tissues, which in this case are located in a specific area of the intestine (Neves, 2015).

The two main categories of diseases that characterise it are CD and UC, which have some overlapping clinical-pathological characteristics and others that are distinct, making a differential diagnosis possible (World Gastroenterology Organisatio Practice Guidelines, 2015).

CD and UC have common clinical and epidemiological characteristics and their causes may be similar (Matos and Figueiredo, 2013).

Below are images of the mucosa of a healthy colon and the differences in the mucosa in the case of CD and UC.

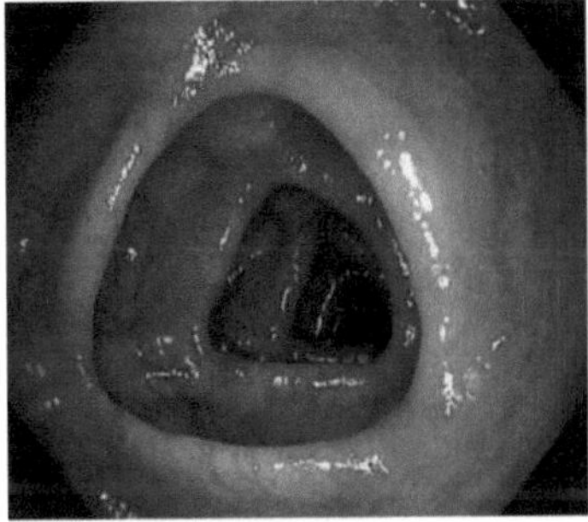
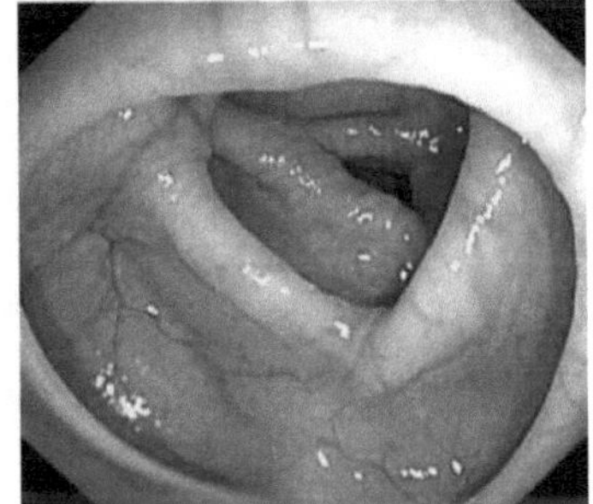

Figure 1 - Images of a healthy colon
Source: http://www.kolumbus.fi/hans/gastrolab/e1009.jpg
Source: http://www.gastrolab.net/ya054h.jpg

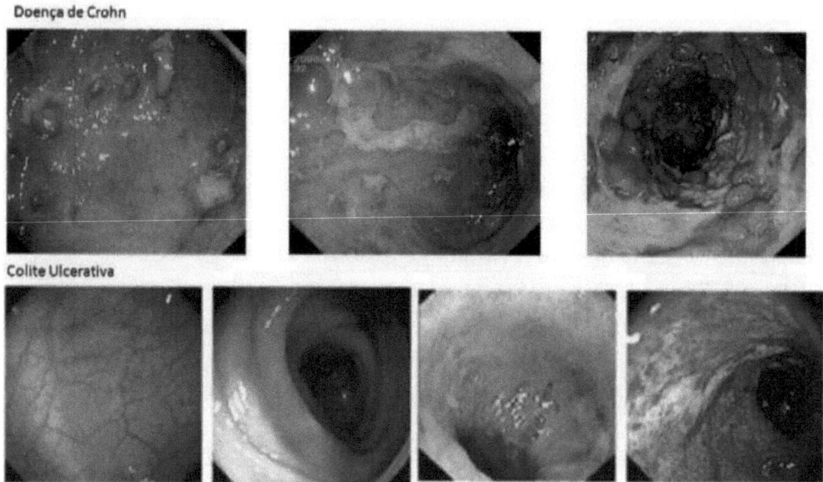

Figure 2 - Images of the differences between DC and CU
Source: http://slideplayer.com.br/slide/10212615/33/images/16/Doen%C3%A7a+of+Crohn+Colitis+Ulcerative.jpg

The incidence of this pathology has been increasing worldwide and is estimated to reach around 0.50 per cent of the population in developed countries, preferably affecting young adults, which will have a significant impact on the QoL of these people, with repercussions at various levels, particularly socially and economically (Matos and Figueiredo, 2013).

The pathogenesis of IBD is not fully understood. Genetic and environmental factors, such as the modification of luminal bacteria and increased intestinal permeability, play an important role in the misregulation of intestinal immunity, which leads to gastrointestinal damage (World Gastroenterology Organisation Practice Guidelines, 2015). Some research shows that IBD can arise due to environmental agents such as pesticides, food additives, tobacco, radiation and non-steroidal anti-inflammatory drugs (Smeltzer et al., 2011).

In addition to CD and UC, IBD includes indeterminate IBD, which, because it has common epidemiological, genetic, immunological, clinical and therapeutic aspects, is included in the same disease.

This pathology has clinical entities of unknown aetiology that are identified with inflammatory lesions on the mucosa of the digestive tract, especially the small intestine and colon.

If the inflammatory lesion is localised only in the mucosa of the colon, with continuous lesions in which ulcers predominate, the disease is called UC. However, if the inflammatory lesion preferentially affects the small intestine and is sometimes associated with discontinuous colon lesions, it is called CD (Quina et al., 2000), as can be seen in the following figure.

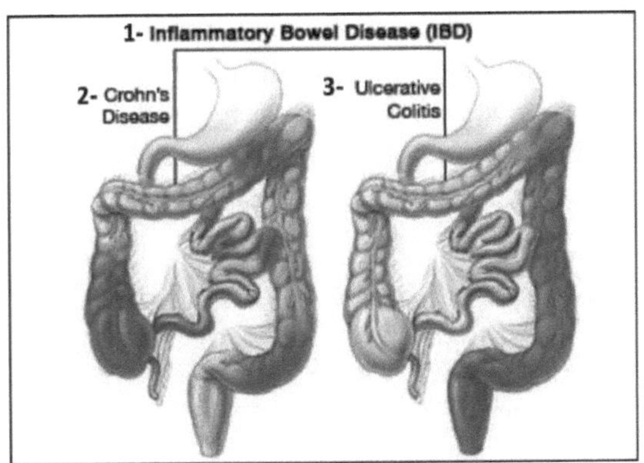

Figure 3 caption
1- Inflammatory Bowel Disease
2- Crohn's disease
3- Ulcerative colitis
Figure 3 - Image of the intestinal localisation of IBD
Source: https://cdn-images-1.medium.com/max/1600/1*ksew41ym-qns4q-doqvb4g.png

IBD is a multifactorial disease in which, faced with an environmental stimulus, a genetically vulnerable host reacts with an uncontrolled immune response. The diagnosis of IBD depends on the results of clinical, radiological, endoscopic and histological examinations. In addition to the lesions in the digestive tract, the different extraintestinal manifestations condition the follow-up and treatment of people (Matos and Figueiredo, 2013), and it is often based on these manifestations that IBD is diagnosed, corresponding to a percentage of 10 to 20 per cent of the diagnoses made (Onal, Yuksel and Bayrakceken, 2015).

People with IBD are at increased risk of osteoporotic fractures as a result of decreased bone density as a result of corticosteroid therapy (Smeltzer et al., 2011), chronic inflammatory activity, intestinal malabsorption and disturbances in circulating levels of sex hormones. These bone alterations will condition people's lives insofar as they have a direct impact on their degree of mobility, promoting greater levels of suffering and fragility and exposing them to the imminent risk of fractures, with a consequent reduction in their QoL. In this sense, there is an urgent need for health professionals to detect, prevent and treat osteoporosis in these people, especially in cases of CD (Lérias, Portela and Pereira, 2000).

In addition to the most common intestinal symptoms such as diarrhoea, intestinal spasms, blood/mucus in the stools, rectal tenesmus and occasional febrile spikes, IBD can reveal itself through a series of extraintestinal manifestations that health professionals sometimes don't associate with the disease. These manifestations can cover various organs or structures, with the most frequent occurring at rheumatological level, particularly in the joints, such as arthralgia and ankylosing spondylitis; at dermatological level, cases of erythema nodosum and psoriasis; at ophthalmological level, cases of uveitis and episcleritis; on a urological level, cases of renal lithiasis, renal failure and nephrosclerosis; on a hepatic and biliary level, cases of cholelithiasis, steatosis and sclerosing cholangitis; on a pulmonary level, cases of pleural effusion, bronchiectasis and asthma; and on a vascular level, cases of venous thrombosis and vasculitis (Torres et al., 2011).

The symptoms experienced by people with IBD can have a major impact on their attitudes and behaviour in life, as well as on emotional, social, physical and sexual aspects (Barros, 2016). It manifests itself in fatigue, pain, shame and, consequently, isolation. In turn, these symptoms can generate negative aspects in the person's life and day-to-day life, interfering on a social, labour and emotional level.

IBD is an intermittent chronic disease that has periods of exacerbation and remission, with the severity of symptoms varying from mild to severe during relapses and many symptoms decreasing or even disappearing during remissions, depending on the segment of the intestinal tract involved (World Gastroenterology Organisation Practice Guidelines, 2015). It usually affects young adults and has a chronic relapsing clinical course, with an impact on health-related quality of life, particularly in aspects related to education, work, social and family life. It is one of the main areas of intervention in gastroenterology (ACSS, 2009).

This disease does not have a specific etiology, although there may be some hereditary relationship when several cases occur in the same family, and it always manifests itself during periods when the person is experiencing high levels of *stress* (Neves, 2015).

Among gastroenterological pathologies, we can distinguish between situations with a major social impact that can be dealt with on an outpatient basis and other more serious situations that require hospitalisation, one of which is IBD (ACSS, 2009).

Crohn's disease

CD is usually first diagnosed in adolescents or young adults, but can appear at any age. The etiology of the disease is not yet known, but the most likely hypothesis is the existence of a certain factor (virus, bacteria) that provokes an immunological response in the body. This immune response will subsequently cause inflammation of the intestine, even when the causative agent is no longer present.

CD affects men and women in equal proportions and is more common in some families. However, some studies report a higher incidence in women.

The disease appears with oedema, thickening of the mucosa and the appearance of ulcers on the inflamed mucosa. The lesions are not continuous, but are separated by healthy tissue and take on a classic "parallelepiped" appearance. It is characterised as a subacute and chronic inflammation of the digestive tract with the possibility of causing inflammation deeper in the intestinal wall (transmural), which can occur in any location of the gastrointestinal tract, from the mouth to the anus. Although it can occur throughout the digestive tract, it is most common in the distal ileum and to a lesser extent in the ascending colon, and is characterised by periods of remission and exacerbation of the disease (Smeltzer et al., 2011).

The symptoms presented are diffuse and not very objective, characterised by abdominal pain, more intense in the lower right quadrant, weight loss and diarrhoea, and the pain is not relieved by defecation. As a result of this frequent diarrhoea, health professionals are faced with people who are emaciated, anorectic and with dietary deficits (Smeltzer et al., 2011).

As the disease progresses, the intestinal wall thickens, becoming fibrotic and narrowing the lumen. The affected intestinal loops sometimes join with others that surround them; inflammation can reach the perianal region and extraintestinal manifestations can develop, such as joint disorders, skin lesions, eye disorders and oral ulcers, and abscesses, fistulas and fissures can also appear (Smeltzer et al., 2011; Matos and Figueiredo, 2013).

Complications of this condition include intestinal obstruction or stenosis, which may require surgery, perianal disease, hydroelectrolytic imbalance and malnutrition due to malabsorption. Ulcers can appear in any area of the digestive tract, including the mouth, anus and genital area. Fistulas are also common, when ulcers extend through the wall of the intestine, creating an abnormal connection between two areas of the intestine, between the intestine and the skin or between the intestine and another organ, such as the bladder or vagina (Smeltzer et al., 2011; Matos and Figueiredo, 2013).

The appearance of fistulas, fissures and abscesses has a negative impact on a person's QoL, as they affect their functioning at various levels, such as sex, since people experience pain during sex (dyspareunia), specifically when the fistulas are located between the rectum and vagina (Smeltzer et al., 2011).

Perforation of the intestine can occur due to the inflammatory process, leading to the formation of intra-abdominal and anal abscesses. It is also known that the risk of colon neoplasia is quite high (Smeltzer et al., 2011).

The occurrence of neoplasia in CD is higher in men and it occurs at an earlier age (45 to 50 years), compared to small intestine carcinomas (65 years) (Valério, Cutait, Sipahi, Damião and Leite, 2006).

The risk factors for this type of neoplasm are not yet well defined, but the early onset of IBD and its long evolution may be one of the causes. In the majority of reported cases, the neoplasm develops many years after the onset of symptoms, occurring in 79% of patients 20 years after the onset of CD and in 53% after 30 years (Valério, Cutait, Sipahi, Damião and Leite, 2006).

Nutrition in CD is fundamental, since it can be both a triggering factor and a method of treating the disease. Nutritional support is an integral part of treating these people and should be individualised according to each person's needs, the stage of the disease and food intolerances. Therefore, nutritional therapy must be adjusted to the stage of the disease and the person, ensuring that nutritional needs are met and that there are improvements in symptoms and the progression of mucosal healing (Oliveira, Antunes, Santos, Marques and Sousa, 2017).

There is no way of preventing this pathology, and it is only possible to try to prevent or delay symptomatic crises, so adherence to the therapeutic regime is very important in reducing the risk of the disease worsening (Simão, 2014).

There is a greater tendency for recurrence in smokers, so patients with CD should be advised to stop smoking (Santos, 2015).

Ulcerative colitis

UC can appear at any age, but the most common age group is 15 to 40 and 50 to 80. In 20 per cent of cases, the disease begins during childhood or adolescence and appears equally in men and women.

UC is a chronic IBD with exclusive involvement of the colon and rectum, which is continuous and limited to the mucosa. The rectum is almost always involved and the extent of the disease *is* proximal. Its cause is unknown, however, it is thought that there may be a dysregulation of the immune system of the intestinal mucosa that leads to an exaggerated immune response against the normal intestinal microflora, causing the lesions typical of ulcerative colitis (Matos and Figueiredo, 2013).

This pathology attacks the superficial mucosa of the colon and is characterised by multiple ulcers, diffuse inflammation and desquamation. The mucosa becomes oedematous and inflamed, the lesions are close together, abscesses form and there is an infiltrate in the mucosa and submucosa. The inflammatory process begins in the rectum and progresses along the colon, with the intestine narrowing and thickening due to muscle atrophy and fat deposits (Smeltzer et al., 2011).

In general, UC is characterised by periods of exacerbation and remission, with symptoms including bloody diarrhoea, the elimination of pus and mucus, rectal bleeding and/or urgency to defecate, as well as nocturnal defecation, abdominal pain in the left lower quadrant and intermittent tenesmus. Rectorrhages can be significant or not, leading to pallor, anaemia and fatigue. The person may experience anorexia, weight loss, fever, vomiting, dehydration and cramps, and extraintestinal manifestations are not ruled out (Smeltzer et al., 2011; Matos and Figueiredo, 2013).

The complications of UC are toxic megacolon, perforation or haemorrhage as a result of ulceration; osteoporosis; kidney lithiasis; skin diseases; joints and an increased risk of colon neoplasia. In some cases, surgery is necessary to alleviate the effects of the disease and treat serious complications (Smeltzer et al., 2011).

The treatments available make it possible to improve the complaints associated with UC and keep people symptom-free for long periods of time. This will depend on the severity and extent of the disease, the response to previous treatments and the number and severity of previous flares. In people with severe, very frequent acute attacks or colon lesions with a high neoplastic risk, surgical intervention may be necessary. Ultimately, hospitalisation may be necessary to better control worsening crises (Smeltzer et al., 2011).

Although in the majority of cases UC crises are not serious and respond well to treatment, more serious or fatal situations can arise.

Treatment of Inflammatory Bowel Disease

The diagnosis of IBD in adults requires a thorough physical examination and a detailed analysis of the person's anamnesis. There are a variety of tests that should be carried out such as blood and stool tests, endoscopic examinations, biopsies and imaging studies that help to exclude other causes and confirm the diagnosis (World Gastroenterology Organisation Practice Guidelines, 2015).

As it is a chronic disease, continuous monitoring should be carried out, with the above-mentioned tests being particularly important, especially colonoscopy. The risk of colon cancer is higher in people with involvement of the entire colon and with more than 10 years of disease progression. It is therefore essential to monitor the colon regularly (1 or 2 years) by carrying out a colonoscopy and taking small fragments of mucosa for histological study (Smeltzer et al., 2011).

Despite the differences between CD and UC, both forms of IBD cause similar symptoms. The symptoms arise because the affected part of the intestine doesn't work properly.

Treatment can be pharmacological and/or surgical, depending on the type of disease and its extent. The aims of treatment are to eliminate inflammatory crises, suppress inappropriate immune responses and provide rest for the diseased intestine to facilitate healing of the lesions. At the same time, they aim to relieve symptoms, reduce the need for surgery, prevent future relapses, discontinue the use of corticosteroids and reduce the number of hospitalisations, thus contributing to an improvement in the person's QoL. A large number of people who comply with the therapeutic regime have long periods of improvement in their state of health (Smeltzer et al., 2011; Matos and Figueiredo, 2013).

Symptoms can be relieved with antidiarrhoeal medication, antispasmodics or drugs that help with food absorption, as prescribed by a doctor.

There have been some changes in terms of the treatment of IBD, namely the inclusion of immunomodulatory drugs and the use of biological therapy at an early stage, in order to alter the course of the disease to the detriment of the continued use of steroids (Palmela, Torres and Cravo, 2015).

The most effective treatment is related to the use of new biological therapies and immunosuppressants, so it is advised that people start treatment as early as possible in order to avoid irreversible damage to the digestive tract and thus prevent the loss of intestinal function (Matos and Figueiredo, 2013).

UC has a more stable incidence rate, and in recent years progress has been made in the treatment of IBD, particularly in the use of biological therapy. IBD has a significant economic burden, made worse by hospitalisations and surgical interventions, particularly in CD, with hospitalisation accounting for 80% of total costs. On the other hand, chronic medical therapy only accounts for 10% of total treatment costs (ACSS, 2009).

Surgery is only performed when other measures have not proved effective. The person is indicated for surgery if there is no improvement in their state of health and if there is continued deterioration of the intestine, heavy bleeding, perforation, stenosis formation and, in some cases, neoplasia of the colon. The option of surgical treatment depends on the ineffectiveness of the treatment and the complications that will interfere with the person's QoL. As a rule, surgery tends to improve QoL, and proctocolectomy with ileostomy is recommended. In some more serious situations, especially CD, the procedure of choice is total colectomy and ileostomy (Matos and Figueiredo, 2013).

The person must be aware, well informed and in agreement with the therapeutic option chosen, in order to promote efficient adherence to the therapeutic regime, since it is a chronic disease that requires continuous clinical and pharmacological monitoring for an indefinite period of time (World Gastroenterology Organisation Practice Guidelines, 2015).

Treatment will progressively evolve in stages until the desired response is achieved. The main goal of IBD treatment, in addition to symptom control, is nutritional balance and improving people's QoL (Fróes, 2012).

IBD and its implications often cause changes in dietary intake, either due to a reduction in intake as a result of the gastrointestinal symptoms associated with the disease or due to changes in the absorption of the nutrients ingested.

In the study by Silva, Schieferdecker and Amarante (2011), it was shown that people with this condition, whether in activity or remission, have inadequate food intake. There are some food intolerances, particularly to lactose, vegetables and pulses in general and, in this sense, there has been a reduction in the intake of these foods, since they increase intestinal motility and cause greater discomfort.

Nutritional therapy prescribes a diet appropriate to the person, depending on their pathology, in order to reduce inflammation and control diarrhoea and pain. In people with malabsorption, it may be necessary to administer vitamins and minerals. When necessary, and in cases where the disease is more serious, the person may need to be hospitalised to correct the hydroelectrolytic imbalance, and intravenous therapy may be used (Matos and Figueiredo, 2013).

A person's nutritional status is directly related to the severity of the disease and malnutrition is a complication that hinders prognosis. Nutritional therapy is used to prevent or correct malnutrition, re-establish macro and micronutrient deficits and correct some of the metabolic consequences characteristic of this pathology. In most people, nutritional therapy acts as an adjunct to clinical or surgical treatment, but in some specific situations it can be the main treatment (Santos, Dorna, Vulcano et al., 2015).

The diet of these people should be balanced and unrestricted, so good eating habits should be recommended (Silva et al., 2011).

Alcohol consumption and active and passive exposure to tobacco should be avoided. Sun exposure and physical activity should be promoted, as well as an adequate calcium and vitamin D diet, especially for people taking corticosteroids (Lérias et al., 2000).

1.1.1 - Epidemiological data and aetiology of Inflammatory Bowel Disease

According to epidemiological studies carried out over the last few decades, the incidence of IBD in the world's population has been increasing, which may be related to changes in people's lifestyles (diet, smoking habits, sedentary lifestyle, *stress)* and the possibility of defining diagnoses earlier, due to improvements in complementary diagnostic techniques and tests (Russell, 2000).

The disease affects people with different characteristics such as age, gender, nationality and even socio-economic status. It is relatively common and affects approximately 1.40 million people in the United States, 2.20 million in Europe and around 150,000 people (0.50 per cent) of the population of Canada (Souza, Belasco and Aguilar-nascimento, 2008).

The United States of America, England, Italy, Scandinavia and Northern Europe are considered high incidence countries; the countries of Southern Europe, South Africa, Australia and New Zealand are intermediate incidence countries, and finally Asia, South America and Brazil are low incidence countries (Souza et al., 2008).

In England, the prevalence of CD is around 55 to 140 per 100,000 inhabitants, and UC is around 160 to 240 per 100,000, with a combined incidence of around 13,300 new cases diagnosed each year. In France, the prevalence of IBD is around 110 per 100,000 inhabitants. Studies were carried out in Portugal in 2005/2006, with around 8,000 cases of IBD. Some studies on CD in Europe show a large increase in incidence over the last 50 years, while others report a considerable increase followed by stabilisation (ACSS, 2009).

IBD is a public health problem in several countries. Important studies have shown that its epidemiology, especially since 1980, has shown an increasing trend worldwide. The incidence of the disease has increased in developed countries, with an estimated 50 to 70 cases per 1,000,000 inhabitants per year (Torres et al., 2011).

Although there are inconsistencies in the different epidemiological studies carried out in Europe (Azevedo, Magro, Portela, Lago, Deus and Cotter, 2010), there are comparative studies that show a higher incidence of IBD in this continent compared to North America. Although epidemiological studies in developing countries are scarce, the incidence and prevalence of IBD is increasing over time, especially in Western countries (Ponder and Long, 2013).

In the 1990s, the incidence of CD and UC increased dramatically in Spain, with a greater impact on CD. Central and South America are the last major regions where IBD is still infrequent. However, with increasing industrialisation there is likely to be a significant increase in IBD in some areas of Central and South America over the next 20 years. UC is more common than CD, as evidenced by various studies carried out in Brazil, Uruguay and Puerto Rico. In Brazil and Mexico, UC has been on the rise, as has CD in Brazil (Farrukh and Mayberry, 2014).

When IBD is diagnosed for the first time in a population, UC precedes CD and has a higher incidence, with a few exceptions, such as Canada and Australia. The annual incidence of UC in Europe varies between 0.60% and 24.30% in 100,000 inhabitants, in Asia and the Middle East it varies between 0.10% and 6.30% in 100,000 inhabitants and in North America it varies between 0 and 19.20% in 100,000 inhabitants. The annual incidence of CD in Europe varies between 0.30 per cent and 12.70 per cent of 100,000 inhabitants; in Asia and the Middle East it varies between 0.04 per cent and 5.00 per cent of 100,000 inhabitants and in North America it varies between 0 and 20.20 per cent of 100,000 inhabitants. The highest prevalence of IBD was observed in Europe, with 505 out of 100,000 inhabitants for UC and 322 out of 100,000 inhabitants for CD. In North America, there were 249 out of 100,000 inhabitants for UC and 319 out of 100,000 inhabitants for CD (Molodecky, Soon, Rabi et al., 2012).

Studies highlighting the temporal patterns of IBD report an increase in incidence in various regions of the globe over the last fifty years (Cosnes, Gower- Rousseau, Seksik, and Cortot, 2011).

As countries become more developed and industrialised, the incidence of UC increases, followed by CD, as has happened in Japan, Singapore and South Korea. In Africa, Central America and South America, data is scarce or unavailable (Cosnes et al., 2011). Industrialisation is associated with a number of potential environmental risk factors for IBD, such as increased exposure to microorganisms, changes in sanitary conditions, changes in diet and lifestyles, taking medication and frequent exposure to pollutants (Molodecky et al., 2012).

A high prevalence of IBD has been observed in Jews, including Jews who emigrated to areas with a low prevalence of the disease. Another study reported a low incidence of IBD in Jews born in Africa, Asia and Israel, compared to Jews born in Europe and North America (Cosnes et al., 2011). These data support the combination of genetic and environmental factors in the genesis of IBD.

The prevalence of IBD in Portugal was assessed through a study of people using anti-inflammatory therapy to treat their pathology, carried out between 2003 and 2007, from which the following conclusions stand out (Azevedo, et al., 2010):

✓ *The* prevalence of IBD almost doubled from 2003 to 2007 (increase in IBD prevalence from 86 to 146 per 100,000 inhabitants, with CD increasing from 43 to 73 per 100,000 inhabitants and UC from 42 to 71 per 100,000 inhabitants from 2003 to 2007);

✓ The prevalence of UC was highest in the 40-64 age group, while CD peaked in the 17-39 age group;

✓ This increase was considerable in all of Portugal's districts, and no distribution pattern (north-south gradient) was confirmed;

✓ The districts with the highest incidence of IBD were Lisbon and Porto (173 and 163 per 100,000 inhabitants respectively). The districts of Castelo Branco and Beja also had a high incidence (> 150 per 100,000 inhabitants).

This study reveals that Portugal is in the middle of the table between high and low incidence countries. IBD has been increasing considerably, perhaps due to the fact that lifestyles have undergone significant changes, namely the abandonment of the Mediterranean diet, which was traditional and offered advantages in achieving a healthy life.

As is the case in other Western countries, the incidence and prevalence of gastroenterological diseases in Portugal is high, which means that there is an increased need for human and technical resources. It is estimated that at least 30 per cent of the European population is affected by a digestive disease at least once in their lives. According to some recent studies, the prevalence of IBD in Portugal is 150 per 100,000 inhabitants, with a tendency to increase progressively (Rede Nacional de Especialidade Hospitalar e de Referenciação, 2016).

In the 1990s, the first epidemiological investigation was carried out at European level, studying the evolution of IBD in Portugal and in various European countries. It was found that the incidence of the disease was 5 per 100,000 inhabitants in the district of Braga and 2 per 100,000 inhabitants in the municipality of Almada. A more recent study, in collaboration with the Inflammatory Bowel Disease Study Group (GEDII), found an incidence of 11 per 100,000 inhabitants. This means that the incidence of these diseases doubled between 1993 and 2012. In another study carried out between 2003 and 2007, the increase in the number of cases was considerable, with an estimated prevalence of IBD of 140 patients per 100,000 inhabitants. These figures suggest that there are around 18,000 IBD sufferers in Portugal (Inflammatory Bowel Disease Study Group, 2017).

This pathology affects around 15,000 to 20,000 Portuguese, most of them young and active, which has a major impact on society. Some cases can be treated on an outpatient basis and other, more serious situations require more specific treatment with hospitalisation. In order to assess the clinical and economic impact on the organisation and provision of Gastroenterology Services, a survey of digestive diseases was carried out by United European Gastroenterology in spring 2013 in 28 countries of the European Union, Norway, Switzerland, Liechtenstein and Russia. The aim was to gather all the available evidence and put into perspective the consequences for health, the burden in terms of public health and to ensure that efforts are prioritised where they are most needed. The study revealed that there is an increase in the incidence of most digestive diseases in Europe, including IBD, with implications for future healthcare provision. IBD, among other digestive diseases, has a major impact on QoL, productivity at work and absenteeism (Rede Nacional de Especialidade Hospitalar e de Referenciação, 2016).

IBD is more common in Caucasians, between the ages of 20 and 40, with a second peak from the age of 55 and a similar distribution in both genders, with the exception of CD, which affects the female population more. The peak age of CD incidence occurs in the third decade of life and the incidence rate decreases with age. The incidence rate of UC is fairly stable between the third and seventh decade of life (World Gastroenterology Organisation Practice Guidelines, 2015).

The prevalence of CD is higher in urban areas than in rural areas, and is also higher in higher socioeconomic classes, smokers and first-degree relatives (World Gastroenterology Organisation Practice Guidelines, 2015). Epidemiological data can provide information on the natural history of the disease and its complications, help assess public health costs and plan appropriate care for these people (Souza et al., 2008).

It should be noted that in the population that migrates from an area with a low incidence to an area with a higher incidence, there will be an increase in the incidence of IBD (Azevedo et al, 2010). The emigration of young adolescents to developed countries, which belong to a population with a low incidence, will show a higher incidence of IBD, particularly for the first generation of these families who will be born in a country with a high incidence (World Gastroenterology Organisation Practice Guidelines, 2015).

One reason that explains the difference in incidence between developed and developing nations is related to hygiene issues, since people who are less exposed to childhood infections or unhygienic conditions lose beneficial micro-organisms to strengthen the immune system. Another possible reason for the onset of IBD in developing countries is the shift to Western diet and lifestyle (World Gastroenterology Organisation Practice Guidelines, 2015).

As already mentioned, IBD is a chronic and highly debilitating disease that mainly affects young people. The fact that there is no real knowledge of its causal agents makes its prevention difficult. There is still no cure for this condition, and it has an associated risk of developing into an intestinal neoplasm. In this context, it is essential that the health professionals involved in treatment outline urgent action strategies in clinical practice to prevent the onset of inflammatory crises, guaranteeing sustained control of the disease, preventing future relapses and, in this way, contributing to promoting the QoL of people with this pathology.

Having contextualised the issue of people with IBD, it is now important to address quality of life.

CHAPTER 2

2 - QUALITY OF LIFE

From the above description, it was concluded that inflammatory bowel disease has a negative impact on a person's quality of life.

In this context, it is necessary to address QoL in this chapter, in order to conceptualise it, using various authors and framing it in the context of health and the person with IBD. The importance of the nurse's role in promoting the QoL of these people is also emphasised.

2.1 - CONCEPTUALISING QUALITY OF LIFE

The concept of QoL is relatively recent, dating back to the 60s. It has been the subject of many studies aimed at defining it and finding a scientific way of assessing it (Gonçalves, 2010). It can be considered subjective, dynamic and individual, covering the physical, psychological, social and spiritual dimensions. It translates the degree or state of superiority conferred on someone or something, and the concept of life covers the condition of a person's complete functional activity, taking into account their behaviour, development, sources of pleasure or suffering and their lifestyle in general (Canavarro and Vaz Serra, 2010).

For Minayo, Hartz and Buss (2000), this concept is particularly human and resembles the degree of satisfaction found in family, love, social and environmental life and existence itself. It depends on the ability to realise a cultural summary of all the elements that a given society considers to be its standard of comfort and well-being.

The aforementioned authors ensure that non-material values such as love, freedom, happiness, solidarity, social inclusion and personal fulfilment are also associated with this concept.

The term QoL includes many meanings, which reflect the knowledge, experiences and values of people and groups who refer to it at different times, in different spaces and in different histories (Minayo et al., 2000).

Although there are various attempts to define QoL, there is no concept that is fully accepted, as it not only includes factors related to health, such as physical, functional, emotional and mental well-being, but also other important elements in people's lives such as: work, material conditions, housing, relationships, family, friends, happiness, love and freedom. It is a holistic concept that encompasses multiple meanings, reflecting individual and collective knowledge, experiences and values.

As can be seen, there are different variables that influence QoL, including current lifestyle, previous experiences, life goals and expectations, support system and level of *stress at* work (Gonçalves, 2010).

Canavarro and Vaz Serra (2010), based on the WHO definition, state that QoL corresponds to each person's perception of their position in life, without neglecting the context of the physical, cultural and social environment in which they are integrated, according to their goals, expectations, concerns and life models.

According to Campolina, Dini and Ciconeli (2011), QoL translates the individual assessment that each person makes of their life, of their state of health, taking into account the various domains of human nature, namely: physical, psychological, emotional, social, spiritual, economic, among others.

QoL is currently an elementary topic of research in the health area, since its results contribute to the approval and definition of the type of treatments to be implemented and, consequently, the evaluation of the cost/benefit of the care provided (Dantes, Sawada and Malerbo, 2003). It consists of the person's perception between real life and their own expectations, taking into account the fulfilment of their goals and dreams. Thus, among the many different factors that can influence people's QoL, there is a particular emphasis on aspects related to health (Vintém, 2008).

QoL assessment is becoming part of clinical practice in order to identify problems that interfere with people's well-being and lives, and is an effective measure for the therapeutic assessment of people and groups of people (Anes and Ferreira, 2009). In this sense, it represents a way of quantifying, in scientific and analysable terms, the consequences of the disease and its treatment, according to the person's perception, seeking to know what conditions their QoL (Costa, Tavares, Trindade and Dias, 2012).

From a subjective perspective, the assessment of QoL depends directly on the person's assessment. In the multidimensional domain, it is important to assess physical well-being, functional capacity, psychological and social health (Canavarro and Vaz Serra, 2010).

The absence of disease alone does not translate into the notion of QoL. What is required is a dynamic and more comprehensive view of each person's needs, not forgetting that they experience constant processes of change, which constitutes a permanent challenge in the search for, development and implementation of health-promoting strategies.

In this context, the importance of studies on this subject should be highlighted, specifically in their contribution to identifying the specific needs of people throughout their life cycle and as a stimulus for change and the adoption of healthy behaviours.

Bearing in mind that health is an important factor in quality of life, the quality of life in the context of health is discussed below.

2.2 - HEALTH-RELATED QUALITY OF LIFE

Due to the subjective nature of the perception of QoL, the influence of various factors and the multidimensionality that characterises it, not limited to the type of illness diagnosed, the concept of health-related quality of life (HRQoL) and a significant number of assessment instruments for it have emerged.

These instruments are designed to transform subjective information into objective information that can be analysed in a quantifiable way.

The instruments used to assess HRQoL usually have questions organised into groups and aim to obtain specific information on certain aspects that affect people's health and well-being (Noronha, Martins, Dias, Silveira, Paula and Haikal, 2016). These instruments can be applied to any healthy or sick person, regardless of the type of illness. Being multidimensional, they provide a global value, based on the principle that the concept of health and QoL is multifactorial and has a unique value.

There is thus a more generic and comprehensive concept of QoL, which includes health as one of its elements, and the concept of HRQoL, which differs from the former due to its specificity and emphasis on health-related aspects (Praça, 2012).

The concept of health for the aforementioned author, compared to QoL, is now considered to be subjective, dynamic and associated with positive aspects, emphasising the importance of social, environmental, economic and educational conditions, with the biological component no longer being highlighted. The growing importance of QoL in the area of health is due to the search for greater well-being for the population and, consequently, the need to define and improve health promotion strategies.

HRQoL translates a state of health, centred on the subjective evaluation of the person, which is directly related to the impact on the person's ability to live fully (Pires, 2009). It can therefore be seen as the value attributed to life, weighted by functional damage, perceptions and social conditions induced by the disease, treatments and the political and economic organisation of the care system (Campos and Neto, 2008).

The term HRQoL is used for a similar purpose to QoL. However, the latter has a broader meaning, manipulated by sociological studies, without necessarily referring to illness and damage, while HRQoL refers to aspects related to illness or health interventions (Canuto, Nogueira and Araújo, 2016), translating a specific concept of the healthcare system, which can be perceived in a general way in the healthy population or according to each disease.

In view of the increase in average life expectancy, various studies have been carried out into the QoL of people suffering from chronic illnesses, in order to find out how the person/family manages to deal with the implications of the illness in their day-to-day lives.

For a better understanding of this subject, we will now look at the Quality of Life of People with Chronic Illness, namely Inflammatory Bowel Disease.

2.3 - QUALITY OF LIFE FOR PEOPLE WITH CHRONIC ILLNESS - INFLAMMATORY BOWEL DISEASE

Each person reacts to a disease situation in a very personal and subjective way, whether in physical, psychological or emotional terms. Because IBD is a chronic pathology, it can cause endless problems for people, resulting from the treatment, which is not always effective, and the associated psychological changes, with direct repercussions on the QoL of the person/family (Mowat, Cole, Windsor et al., 2011).

IBD has significant implications for people's QoL, with levels varying depending on whether the disease is in the active phase or in remission. In the more active phase, the effects of intestinal symptoms on people's lives are visible, and consequently on their ability to fulfil their activities of daily living, leisure and work. However, it is also clear that the QoL levels of these people in remission are always lower when compared to the QoL levels of a normally healthy person (Trindade, Ferreira and Gouveia, 2016).

A person involved in a process of illness is subject to significant changes in their life plans in the short, medium and long term, with inherent changes in their habits, customs and behaviours in association with new ways of thinking and acting (Molodecky and Kaplan, 2010).

There has been a great deal of investment in developing techniques and strategies to deal with IBD. The aim is to alter the natural course of this disease, avoiding as much as possible the inherent intestinal damage and the impact on the QoL of those affected by this pathology (Palmela et al., 2015).

Although there are numerous studies on QoL, when it comes to IBD specifically, the existing studies are scarce and relatively recent. Knowing the impact this disease has on people's lives, it's important to know how their QoL is affected and in what areas, in order to ensure the correct and timely development of wellbeing-promoting strategies.

In this context, assessing the perception of the QoL of people with IBD is essential in order to promote its improvement and understand its influence on their state of health, and it is essential to use measuring instruments adapted and validated for this specific type of population, which is an important factor in optimising treatment for these people (Costa et al., 2012).

IBD causes physical, psychological and social changes that have a strong impact on people's ability to carry out their activities of daily living independently and without limitations, as it is characterised by frequent hospitalisations and prolonged treatments. Since IBD is a chronic disease characterised by periods of stagnation or greater activity, it follows that its impact on people's QoL is significant (Magalhães et al., 2015).

The existence of complications in the intestinal and extraintestinal tract lead to various psychosocial and economic problems associated with school and work absenteeism, depressive states, altered body image and low self-esteem, difficulties in socialisation and sexuality, difficulties with eating, fear of going out and not finding a toilet available, among others, negatively influencing the perception of QoL (Santos,

Silva and Santana, 2014).

People say they have problems with their diet and are therefore often diagnosed with nutritional deficits, which lead to anaemia and delayed growth, as well as systemic complications. Nutritional disorders represent a public health problem that can affect people from any social class (Santos, Silva and Santana, 2014).

In the study carried out by Sarlo, Barreto and Domingues (2008) with people with CD, it was concluded that the impact of this disease was mainly in terms of the changes they suffer in their personal life project, as they are faced with the need to modify their habits, customs and behaviours, especially in terms of diet and the emotional component, not excluding the efforts made to cope with the physical changes resulting from the disease.

In more detail and according to the analysis of the interviews carried out, the aforementioned authors conclude that people reveal two distinct ways of coping with their illness process:

1. Related to the complications inherent in the disease (food, pain, transmission to offspring, relational changes in the family, chronicity of the disease and limited sense of freedom).
2. Related to the need to change behaviours, assuming a positive character, specifically in changing eating habits, practising physical exercise and adopting behaviours to prevent complications, maintaining an optimistic attitude towards the future and the hope of a cure.

These people find it difficult to change their eating habits because they feel frustrated that they can no longer eat the foods they used to love and are forced to follow a specific, restrictive diet. Some don't eat enough food for fear of suffering pain and gastrointestinal changes, while others are well-informed and know how to identify the foods that cause them discomfort and are able to eliminate them from their diet (Sarlo et al., 2008).

The food issue is also reflected in social relationships, as the frequency of social dinners is restricted, which generates feelings of discouragement as it implies the exclusion of some social events and rituals that have been part of their lives for long periods of time (Sarlo et al., 2008).

Still referring to the aforementioned study, the authors conclude that the issue of self-image and the changes that have taken place cause people discomfort, as they no longer feel attractive due to the surgeries and weight loss that characterise this disease, which will affect them emotionally.

Having a chronic illness and the connotation of being chronically ill makes people feel more inferior and with low self-esteem, promoting relational changes and awakening feelings of guilt for not making their partner happy or even in relationships with other people, which can lead to processes of loneliness and suffering, which will be damaging on a psychological and emotional level (Sarlo et al., 2008).

For the younger population, the fear of not being able to follow through with their life plans is evident, specifically with regard to starting a family.

The instability that characterises this disease, mediated by the periods of activity and remission that characterise it, causes anxiety in people, making them fragile, vulnerable and anxious about the future, in terms of prognosis and well-being. They tend to find mechanisms to help overcome the difficulties inherent in experiencing a chronic illness. Often the search involves self-analysis, discovering their own resources, which facilitates behavioural change, the adoption of healthier lifestyles and the attribution of greater meaning and significance to life (Sarlo et al., 2008).

QoL is seen as an individual and diligent judgement. In order to achieve optimum or acceptable levels, it is necessary to develop attitudes to health and illness, i.e. to consider each person as a whole so that we can intervene to prevent illness and promote health. In this sense, it should be viewed in accordance with the person's perception, taking into account a diversity of conditions that encompass their feelings and behaviours, and not limited to their clinical situation (Costa et al., 2012).

The main objective of the studies that have focused on QoL is to determine the impact of the illness on people's lives, identifying support needs and the action to be taken to fulfil them (Costa et al., 2012).

Studies carried out in this area are useful in that they allow us to look at the person holistically and develop more appropriate strategies and approaches aimed at the continuous monitoring of these patients (Magalhães et al., 2015).

Some studies have shown that IBD is on the increase worldwide and as such should be seen as a public health problem, making it essential to know how to minimise the discomfort and complications associated with this disease, so that the large number of people with IBD can have the best possible QoL, avoiding absenteeism from work and consecutive hospitalisations.

Experiencing IBD can condition people to have feelings and emotions that threaten their well-being, leading them to adopt avoidance and evasion behaviours that don't help them cope with the disease.

Developing strategies to cope with this pathology has proved essential for people to demonstrate better levels of well-being, adaptation and acceptance of the disease (Trindade, Ferreira and Gouveia, 2016). It is important to realise the impact of the disease on the daily life of the person/family, in order to promote conditions that help them to experience this disease process, leading to increased well-being and satisfaction for all those involved in order to improve their QoL.

Existing research reveals changes in the QoL of people with IBD, so nursing professionals need to realise the importance of creating conditions aimed at improving it, as can be seen below.

2.4 - THE ROLE OF THE SPECIALIST NURSE IN PROMOTING THE QUALITY
OF LIFE OF PEOPLE WITH CHRONIC ILLNESS - INFLAMMATORY
BOWEL DISEASE

The changes that have taken place in people's health, particularly the increase in chronic diseases, pose challenges for health professionals.

Quality in healthcare is the provision of accessible and equitable healthcare, with professional excellence. With the resources available, health professionals seek citizen adherence and satisfaction and the adaptation of health care to their needs and expectations with a view to the best possible performance (Directorate-General for Health, 2015).

Health education is essential and therefore means creating the conditions for obtaining the necessary information and skills, enabling healthy choices and the transformation of risk behaviours. Change occurs when, in the process of health education, the interests and needs of the person/family and community are valued, involving them as active and participating subjects. This whole process requires dynamic health planning (OE, 2011b).

Nursing's contribution is increasingly important and essential in improving the health of communities, based on the implementation of interventions aimed at health promotion and education (Machado, 2013). In today's world, the community is increasingly aware of its responsibilities in terms of health promotion and, as such, wants to adopt a proactive and partnership role with health professionals, with the aim of improving their well-being and QoL (OE, 2011a).

The Code of Ethics stipulates that all nurses must work in the area of information through health education, encouraging people's independence and autonomous performance. In this way, nurses play a significant role in health promotion and education, always ensuring the active participation of citizens. Health education is an ally for changing behaviour if it is considered a structured citizenship task, designed early on by health professionals. It aims to empower people to take an active role in their health. Thus, one of its main objectives is to help people develop their decision-making capacity and take responsibility for their health (OE, 2011a).

It's important to emphasise the idea that health promotion is about empowering people to be healthy, and that the role of health promoters should encompass the way people define their health goals, thereby helping them to achieve them (Laverack, 2008).

The role of the nurse, as an active element in the health planning process, focuses on identifying the specific learning needs of the community, estimating their concerns. A health education programme is something dynamic and negotiable, which can change according to new needs and situations that arise during its implementation (OE, 2011b).

The WHO argues that it is essential to empower people to learn throughout their lives, preparing them for all stages of their development and to fight against the chronic illnesses and disabilities they may face. These interventions should take place in various contexts, such as school and work (OE, 2011b).

Nurses, as part of a multidisciplinary team, should aim to continuously improve the quality of their care, whether for the person/family or the community, throughout their entire life cycle, with the aim of achieving more and better health for the population (OE, 2011c).

The multidisciplinary team that cares for people will have to consider not only the biological and physical aspects, but also the psychosocial repercussions of the illness. One of the main aims of healthcare is to restore their QoL, in the sense that it is essential for people/families experiencing a chronic illness process (Gimenes, 2013).

QoL, being an individual and subjective concept, depends on their perception of life and the action of various factors such as beliefs, expectations and everything inherent in the treatment and control of their chronic illness. The work of nurses, as they are the health professionals who are most present and closest to the person/family as they experience this whole process, will have a significant influence on the QoL of these people, to the extent that, combined with their knowledge of being, being and their scientific, technical and relational skills, they ensure the satisfaction of the care needed for better well-being.

In the redefinition and qualification of professionals in the face of new challenges, there has been a reconfiguration of the traditional role of nurses towards new trends. In the United States, Canada, New Zealand and the United Kingdom, "Nurses Practitioners" have emerged, who take on some therapeutic prescriptions and diagnostic tests; in Germany, "Community Nurses" who, with some similarity to the previous countries, ensure the provision of primary health care through home visits, especially in rural areas; "Liaison Nurses" in some European countries, particularly the United Kingdom, are responsible for caring for and accompanying people on their return home, in rehabilitation processes, monitoring medication management, education and guidance in relevant situations. Progress in nursing points to an advanced practice, focussed on economic aspects and disease control, rather than on human responses to life and health-disease processes. The vast majority of people with chronic illnesses have difficulties assimilating therapeutic recommendations and integrating them into their daily lives. This phenomenon is related to factors intrinsic to the subjects, but also to a professional practice that does not value people's knowledge of life processes and transitions. As such, nurses must look for action strategies that are effective in caring for people with chronic illnesses and their families (Bastos, 2013).

The increase in the number of people with chronic illnesses in the Portuguese population is a worrying reality, mainly due to its social, economic and, especially, health consequences. Nurses must contribute to improving the population's health by taking preventative action to prevent complications and promote health. This expansion is directly associated with the processes of industrialisation, urbanisation, economic development and food globalisation, which are a set of factors that influence changes in eating habits and promote, for example, sedentary lifestyles, obesity, an increase in addictive habits and, not least, the triggering of worrying *stress* situations (OE, 2010b).

The importance of the role of nurses specialising in community health nursing is clear in the monitoring and care of people with chronic illnesses, effectively contributing to a reduction in the number of medical consultations and the need for hospitalisations, as Sarlo et al. (2008) showed in their study in the United States of America, in which they obtained objective data in this area, specifically a 40.00% reduction in medical consultations and a 20.00% reduction in hospitalisations.

People with chronic illnesses, as well as their families, need a broad level of support to maintain a better state of health. As a rule, these people lack the self-care skills to manage problems at home, so there needs to be care planning to detect any changes in their condition in advance, so that a solution can be found quickly and an acute situation can be avoided (OE, 2010b).

Demographic changes, related to the ageing of the population and the increase in chronic diseases, as well as the current socio-economic and political context contribute to the prospect of nursing care progressing in order to respond to people's new health needs. Nurses provide care centred on the sick person/family and help them to recognise, verbalise and find the most effective way to respond to their health condition, and they are therefore committed to actively managing their illness (Sousa, Martins and Pereira 2015).

The position of the International Council of Nurses (ICN) on the subject of "Informed Patients" considers community participation to be fundamental, attaching fundamental importance to information, as it is a determining factor in decision-making. Nurses should integrate the nature, quality and impact of people's information on health outcomes and nursing practice into their research. In celebration of Nurses' Day (12 May 2010), the ICN launched a worldwide appeal to nurses to lead the fight against chronic disease. They suggested that nurses should be role models for adopting behaviours that protect communities from chronic disease. This call was accompanied by a publication to sensitise nurses to primary and secondary prevention in chronic disease and to increase their proactivity in acquiring new skills and innovation (Bastos, 2013).

Within the scope of the Nursing Care Quality Standards, the Nursing Council (2001) states that one of the functions of nurses is to provide care to healthy or sick people, with the aim of preserving, progressing or regaining their health, enabling them to reach their peak of physical and mental well-being and maximum independence in activities of daily living. Nursing care always takes into account the physical, emotional and social needs of the person/population throughout the life cycle, not forgetting: health promotion, disease prevention, treatment, rehabilitation and social reintegration (OE, 2001).

Caring is essential in nursing and aims to protect, improve and preserve human dignity, by defining values, producing knowledge and developing caring actions, being related to human needs and interconnected with the health-disease binomial (Watson, 2002).

Nursing has evolved as a profession and a discipline, but there is still some reluctance to favour a person-centred approach in practice, as the current care paradigm tends to overvalue the curative aspect (WHO, 2008).

Nursing training is fundamental, and we must invest in training professionals in the factors that influence health behaviours. There is a need to use intervention models that direct nursing practice towards more specific care, in order to support the patient/family in acquiring the skills that will enable them to make informed decisions, becoming more autonomous in managing their health and thus empowering them to take care of their health problems. Although there is a reluctance to change, nurses believe that many of the changes are brought about by the professionals who work in the context of clinical practice, as they continually try to encourage them to adopt lifestyles that are more favourable to their condition, with a view to improving healthcare and, consequently, improving well-being and QoL (Sousa et al., 2015).

Nursing has developed as a discipline, science and art of caring for others, contributing to the provision of quality care with national and international visibility. Nurses are health professionals who take on a decisive and increasingly proactive role in identifying the needs of the population and promoting and protecting people's health, looking at them holistically. Nursing care is essential in the health system, which has its repercussions at regional and national level. It is therefore a theme that needs to be continually developed, involving professionals from all areas of care provision and jointly seeking new meanings about its essence (Backes, Backes, Erdmann and Buscher 2012).

Although nursing is complemented by other professional knowledge, it can be strongly praised and defined as the science of comprehensive and integrative health care, both in terms of assisting and coordinating care practices and promoting and protecting the health of people, families and communities, offering the opportunity to work creatively and autonomously at different levels of health, promoting or rehabilitating the health of communities (Backes et al., 2012).

The role of the nurse is recognised by their capacity and ability to understand the human being in a holistic way, by the comprehensiveness of health care, by their ability to welcome and identify the needs and expectations of people/families, by their ability to accept and understand social differences, and by their ability to promote interaction and association between people, the health team, the family and the community. Nursing seeks to create an effective relationship with the person, regardless of their economic, cultural or social conditions, i.e. it aims to optimise health care interventions in a way that integrates and takes into account both professional knowledge and the information characteristic of people and the community (Backes et al., 2012).

In Neves' opinion,

> For users, the nurse's role was unclear, but their performance exceeded expectations in terms of both technical skills and relational, communicational and cultural skills. Proximity, the ability to listen, to guide, to explain and to provide more detailed information that was framed in the users' social environment, were perceived as interventions that met their needs more adequately (Neves, 2012 p. 132).

The specialist nurse has more in-depth knowledge in a specific area of nursing, not forgetting human responses to life processes and health problems, demonstrating high levels of clinical judgement and decision-making, translated into a set of specialised skills relating to a field of intervention (OE, 2011d).

The care provided by nurses specialising in community and public health nursing must be based on scientific evidence, which is why nursing research is a powerful means of answering questions about people's needs, pressing healthcare interventions and facilitating the definition of better ways of promoting health, preventing illness and providing care and services in the different areas of activity to the person/family, throughout the life cycle and in different contexts (OE, 2011a).

Nurse specialists must have competences in the field of continuous quality improvement. They must play a driving role in developing and supporting institutional strategic initiatives in the area of clinical governance; design, manage and collaborate in continuous quality improvement programmes; create and maintain a therapeutic and safe environment (OE, 2011d).

For Stanhope and Lancaster (2010), intervention in the community is a necessity that meets the origins of community nursing practice, which are the health of individuals, families and groups. Community-oriented practice seeks healthy changes in favour of the community, integrating it as the target of nursing, the collective, the common good, without neglecting individual health, as they coexist.

Community and public health nursing develop a globalised practice centred on the community. The demographic changes felt in society, such as population ageing, morbidity indicators and the occurrence of chronic diseases, show the shortcomings in health. In recent years, primary healthcare has played a decisive role in creating a strong and active society. As a result, nurses specialising in Community and Public Health Nursing, with their knowledge, experience and clinical expertise, develop the capacity to respond to the varied needs felt by people, groups or communities, providing health gains (OE, 2011e).

Community and public health nurses must actively participate in different situations, guaranteeing access to efficient, constant and adapted healthcare, especially for social groups with specific needs (OE, 2011e).

Their practice is based on the regulations governing the specific competences of nurses specialising in community and public health nursing. They contribute to the process of empowering groups and communities by working in partnership with other health professionals and articulating knowledge from the sciences, research, communication and education. They promote health education, the re-establishment, co-ordination, management and evaluation of care for individuals, families and the community. Health promotion and education strategies are adapted to the characteristics of the community, and it is essential to research and diagnose the risk factors of communities in certain geographical areas, guaranteeing efficient, adjusted and continuous care (OE, 2011e).

In this sense, nurses specialising in community and public health nursing play an essential role in health promotion, as they have the skills to coordinate and implement health projects or programmes covering the different sectors of the community: health, education, social networks, different local authority departments and others, which aim to empower groups and communities. Its functions include the creation and planning of intervention programmes for the prevention, protection and promotion of health, with the aim of recognising people's health needs (OE, 2011a).

It is important for nurses specialising in community health nursing to understand what these people experience and feel, and to adopt a professional conduct in which sympathy and support are present to facilitate the process of adoption and acceptance of the illness by the person/family (Sarlo et al., 2008).

The nursing team must guide people and their families, providing all the necessary information to promote correct adherence to the therapeutic regime established, as well as correct fulfilment of the instructions given regarding diet and physical exercise, in order to develop a more healthy lifestyle (Lopes, 2014).

As part of health education, specialised nurses must enable people and their families to adapt to illness in order to prevent complications and solve problems when faced with new realities. The aim of health education is to teach people/families how to live healthier lives, assessing the responsibility that each person has in maintaining/promoting their own health. It is the duty of the members of the healthcare team, more specifically the specialist nurses, to make this education consistent and available. Educational environments can include homes, hospitals, health centres, workplaces, service organisations, shelters and training sessions in health services.

At national level, in 1999, the Ministry of Health defined nursing consultation as an autonomous activity, based on scientific methodologies, where the nurse makes a nursing diagnosis based on the recognition of health needs in general and nursing needs in particular, draws up and implements a care plan according to the degree of dependence of the person and evaluates the care provided and the corresponding reformulation of nursing interventions (Ministry of Health, 2011).

The nursing consultation, in the glossary of the Family Health Units of 2006, is defined as: "an intervention aimed at carrying out an assessment, establishing a nursing care plan, in order to help the individual achieve maximum self-care capacity" (Ministry of Health, 2006 p. 14), which aims to promote health education, teaching and assessing the knowledge and attitudes of people, in this case with chronic bowel disease.

The National Hospital Speciality and Referral Network (2016) believes that there has to be a continuous commitment to a path that always aims to improve methodologies. Gastroenterology requires the definition of "Gastroenterology Nursing", with specialisation in more specific areas, such as the technical area of Digestive Endoscopy, IBD and Hepatology. It will be necessary to invest in adopting new attitudes, which implies changing mentalities and attitudes in order to promote proper management of human resources and facilitate the provision of excellent care.

Since the person is a universe of possibilities, a careful multidisciplinary approach must be taken, which facilitates the development of a correct diagnosis and the definition of a specific and appropriate treatment plan. In this context, the Inflammatory Bowel Disease Study Group considers it essential to integrate nurses into its action strategy and, as such, they were the first to organise the first Inflammatory Bowel Disease Nursing course, stating that "We want to be pioneers in this differentiation of nurses in IBD" (GEDII, 2017, p. 3).

The specialised nurse must be able to develop a set of specific skills to help and support people with IBD and their families, with the aim of improving their QoL. They must be willing to receive and listen to the concerns of the person with IBD / family, accompany them at an early stage of the disease to identify their individual needs and help meet them, providing information about the disease and contacts with other people with IBD and support groups (GEDII) to share doubts and obtain clarification about the disease process.

These health professionals should be the link between the doctor, the person with IBD/family and the rest of the multidisciplinary team so that, together, they can empower the person with IBD and their family to make the right decisions in order to improve their QoL.

People with IBD are part of a group with specific needs and who need to be monitored. Effective healthcare and the development of intervention programmes and projects should be ensured, with a view to empowering them at an individual, family and community level.

In view of the above, it is of great interest to study the problem of the "Perception of the Quality of Life of People with Inflammatory Bowel Disease", with a view to improving it.

The methodological phase of the study is presented below.

CHAPTER 3
EMPIRICAL STUDY

3 - RESEARCH METHODOLOGY

The fundamental starting point for any research is to select an area of interest and transpose it into a question that can be studied, allowing new knowledge to be obtained on the subject. In this way, and given the interest of the topic, it is considered pertinent to develop an investigation into the Quality of Life of People with Inflammatory Bowel Disease, who are followed up at the Outpatient Clinic of a Local Health Unit in the Centre Region.

According to Fortin, Côté and Filion (2009), research methodologies must adopt different attitudes towards human behaviour and the way of approaching knowledge of phenomena.

The methodology aims to clarify the interest in the strategies, procedures and techniques used and, consequently, to acquire answers and results for the objectives set, translating a rational process and a set of techniques or means that allow the research to be carried out (Fortin et al., 2009).

Any research question is a clear question relating to an area that is to be explored with the aim of obtaining new information. The research questions are the principles on which the research results are based and derive directly from the objective, indicating what the researcher wants to obtain as information (Fortin et al., 2009).

In this sense, a research study arises from an observed or perceived problem and cannot proceed unless the subject to be explored is selected, requiring the fulfilment of certain questions that will guide and delimit the methodological process. In general, the basic elements will be addressed, defining: the research question, the type of study, the study objectives, the study hypotheses, the delimitation of the population and respective sample to be studied, the identification and operationalisation of the variables and the data collection instrument. The data collection strategy, sampling criteria and the basic ethical and formal procedures for carrying out this research will also be explained.

3.1 - RESEARCH QUESTION

The research question stems from the problem under study and the theoretical framework selected, resulting directly from the objective and indicating what the researcher wants to obtain as information (Fortin et al., 2009). Thus, the research question of this study is: What is the perception of the quality of life of people with Inflammatory Bowel Disease?

3.2 - TYPE OF STUDY

The type of study can be considered a guideline for the methodology because it determines its structure. Each type of study has its own characteristics which are reflected throughout the research and which allow the study objectives to be achieved to a greater or lesser extent.

In view of the problem under study, this work falls within the field of descriptive-correlational, cross-sectional and quantitative research.

In a descriptive-correlational study, the aim is to explore relationships between variables and describe them, making it possible to determine which variables are associated with the phenomenon studied (Fortin et al., 2009).

In terms of time, this study can be classified as cross-sectional, since cross-sectional studies aim to assess the frequency of an event or disease and its risk factors in a given population, and the quantitative method is one that "... emphasises explanation and prediction, is based on measuring phenomena and analysing numerical data" (Fortin et al., 2009, p. 27).

3.3 - STUDY OBJECTIVES

According to Fortin et al. (2009), the aim of the research is to clearly and objectively indicate the goal that the researcher is pursuing, to characterise the key variables, the population from which data will be collected and the action verb that will guide the research. For the same authors, the aim of a study "is to describe, explain or predict, according to the state of knowledge in the field studied" (2009, p. 160).

The aim of a research project is to develop or study a new subject or to deepen a subject already developed by other researchers, in order to increase the level of knowledge about it and thus, in the case of the health sciences, to be able to contribute to improving people's well-being and QoL.

The following objectives were therefore set for this study:

1. To assess the perception that people with inflammatory bowel disease have of their quality of life;
2. To analyse the factors that determine the quality of life of people with inflammatory bowel disease;

The aim of this study is to study a group of people with IBD and assess their perception of QoL, correlating the factors that determine it, in order to identify problems and define strategies to improve their QoL.

3.4 - STUDY HYPOTHESES

Formulating research hypotheses is a crucial step in carrying out a research study. These must be clear and logically consistent, requiring the researcher to be original, reflecting on their personal experience, interest and knowledge of the subject to be investigated.

According to Fortin et al. (2009, p.165), a hypothesis "takes into account the key variables and the population" and is a "statement that anticipates relationships between variables and requires empirical verification". The formulation of a hypothesis implies the verification of a theory, or rather its propositions, and includes the problem, the variables under study, the target population and the type of research to be carried out, predicting the results of the studies (Fortin et al., 2009).

According to Fortin et al. (2009), hypotheses influence:

> Research design;
> Data collection and analysis methods;
> Interpretation of results.

In this study, the hypotheses formulated aim to establish a supposed relationship between the variables under study and include:

> **Hypothesis 1** - There is a relationship between the perception of the QoL of people with IBD and sociodemographic variables;
> **Hypothesis 2** - There is a relationship between the perception of the QoL of people with IBD and behavioural habits;
> **Hypothesis 3** - There is a relationship between the perception of the QoL of people with IBD and clinical variables.

3.5 - TARGET POPULATION, SAMPLE AND SAMPLING CRITERIA

The population or universe refers to all the individuals who have the same characteristics defined for a given study (Fortin et al., 2009).

A target population consists of a group of elements or subjects that have common characteristics, according to certain criteria.

According to Fortin (1999), the target population is made up of those who meet the selection criteria defined in advance, which in this case are people with IBD, and for whom the researcher wishes to make generalisations.

The inclusion criteria are the characteristics that delimit the population of interest. It is up to the researcher to establish these criteria before selecting the sample, in order to decide whether or not a person would be classified as a member of the population in question.

The inclusion criteria defined for this study are as follows:

> People registered for outpatient consultations with IBD at a Local Health Unit in the Centre Region;
> Be aged between 18-65;
> Know how to read and write Portuguese;
> Have the cognitive skills to complete the questionnaire; > Agree to take part in the study on a voluntary basis.

The study sample was consecutive by convenience, taking into account the time period established for data collection, which was between January and September 2017.

Using the Epi-Info Version 7 programme, it was possible to calculate the number of members of the sample, based on the target population. In this sense, and knowing that the target population is made up of 155 people, for an estimated frequency of 50%, an acceptable margin of error of 15% and a 95% confidence interval, a sample made up of 33 people should be studied. As the sample in this study is made up of 38 members, it can be judged to have acceptable sampling consistency.

3.6 - OPERATIONALISATION OF VARIABLES

Variables are qualities, properties or characteristics of people, objects or situations that can change or vary over time and usually take on different values that can be measured, manipulated or controlled. Depending on their role in the research, they can be considered independent, dependent or attribute (Fortin et al., 2009).

3.6.1 - Dependent variable

The dependent variable "is the one that suffers the effect of the independent variable" (Fortin et al., 2009, p.171), translating the behaviour, response or result observed as a function of the presence of the independent variable. It is often referred to as the criterion variable or the explained variable (Fortin et al., 2009).

In this study, the dependent variable is:

- Perceived Quality of Life of People with Inflammatory Bowel Disease

3.6.2 - Independent variables

For Fortin et al. (2009), the independent variable is the variable that the researcher manipulates in order to measure its effect on the dependent variable.

The following independent variables were considered in this study: Socio-demographic variables, considering the following as the most important:

- Age;
- Gender;
- Marital status;
- Educational level;
- Profession.
- Age - continuous variable, measurable in years, from birth to the date of data collection.
- Gender - dichotomous variable, which takes the category of female or male.
- Marital status - nominal variable, which takes the category of single, married, divorced or widowed.
- Level of schooling - nominal variable, which assumes five categories: no schooling, fourth grade, 9th grade, 12th grade and higher education.
- Occupation - a nominal variable, which takes on four categories: employed, unemployed, student and retired.

<u>Behavioural habits,</u> in particular:
- ➢ Smoking habits;
- ➢ Alcohol habits.
- ✓ Smoking habits - nominal variable, with three categories: non-smoker, former smoker and smoker.
- ✓ Alcohol habits - nominal variable, with three categories: non-existent, mild and moderate.

<u>Clinical variables,</u> which include:
- ➢ Confirmation of diagnosis;
- ➢ Hospital admissions;
- ➢ Diagnosis time.
- ✓ Confirmation of diagnosis - Crohn's Disease, Ulcerative Colitis and Undetermined Inflammatory Disease;
- ✓ Hospital admissions - dichotomous variable, categorised as yes or no. If the answer is yes, an open question is asked in which the participant mentions the reason for the hospitalisation;
- ✓ Diagnosis time - continuous variable, measured in years.

3.7 - DATA COLLECTION INSTRUMENT

Any research instrument used to carry out a piece of research must enable reliable and relevant information to be collected. The nature of the research problem determines the type of data collection method to be used, and its choice depends on the variables and their operationalisation, as well as the statistical analysis strategy used (Fortin et al., 2009).

The use of self-administered questionnaires has proven to be one of the most widely used ways of collecting data, as it makes it possible to measure what you want more accurately and its impersonal nature helps to ensure uniformity in the evaluation of the data.

In order to carry out this study, data was collected using an instrument made up of two parts. The first consists of a set of questions covering three dimensions: sociodemographic, behavioural and clinical (Appendix A). The second is the *Inflammatory Bowel Disease Questionnaire* (IBDQ-R). This questionnaire was first developed in 1988 in the United States by Mitchell et al. and was later restructured by Guyatt et al. (1988), reducing the original 150 items to the current 32, grouped into 4 dimensions: Intestinal Symptoms; Systemic Symptoms; Emotional Aspects and Social Aspects; with 7 hypothetical answers in which 1 corresponds to the worst levels of quality of life and 7 to the best (Pontes, Miszputen, Fereira, Miranda and Ferraz, 2004).

In this study, the instrument used was translated and validated for the Portuguese population by Veríssimo (1996, 1997). It consists of 32 items with 7 response hypotheses, where 1 corresponds to "normal or never" and 7 to "very much or always", corresponding to better or worse levels of quality of life, respectively.

The questionnaire makes it possible to assess different aspects of QoL, which are grouped into 4 dimensions: Intestinal Symptoms; Systemic Symptoms; Emotional Aspects and Social Aspects (Table 1), addressing questions related to the symptoms people have, how they have been feeling and their state of mind over the last fortnight, allowing us to understand how they have adapted to their illness (Veríssimo, 2008).

This is an abbreviated version, but it shows psychometric properties, since in terms of fidelity this instrument has a Cronbach's Alpha of 0.92 for the total questionnaire and an average of 0.82 for the different sub-scales or dimensions that make it up.

Each question is based on a 7-point *Likert* scale, with positive and negative items taken into account and the corresponding *score* converted. The negative items (inverted items) are 6, 21 and 32.

The fact that it has been readjusted to 32 questions allows it to be reduced to two pages, which makes it easier for participants to fill in in terms of time and practical applicability. All participants are briefly informed before filling in the form, in order to alert them to the need for their answers to refer to aspects and symptoms experienced in the last fortnight/two weeks.

Table 1 - Items per dimension of the IBDQ-R-32 Questionnaire

	Alpha of Cronbach's	Possible *scores*	
		Minino	Maximum
Intestinal symptoms (10 items) Items 01; 05; 09; 13; 17; 20; 22; 24; 26 and 29	0.84	10	70
Systemic Symptoms (5 items) Items 02; 06; 10; 14 and 18	0.77	5	35
Emotional Aspects (12 items) Items 03; 07; 11; 15; 19; 21; 23; 25; 27; 30; 31 and 32	0.87	12	84
Social Aspects (5 items) Items 04; 08; 12; 16 and 28	0.87	5	35

In the total questionnaire (IBDQ-R) we have a minimum *score of* 32 points, which translates into better QoL, and a maximum *score of* 224 points, which translates into worse QoL. Given that there is no QoL assessment according to the *scores that* can be obtained with this questionnaire, we opted for a cut-off point classification. In this sense, the QoL perceived by people with IBD was classified as follows:

✓ *Score* 0-20 - Poor QoL;

✓ *Score* 20-40 - Poor QoL;

✓ *Score* 40-60 - Fair QoL;

✓ *Score 60-80* - Good QoL;

✓ *Score* 80-100 - Excellent QoL.

3.8 - ETHICAL AND DATA COLLECTION PROCEDURES

In research involving data on human beings, ethics and deontology must be strictly respected. Before carrying out a study, the researcher should ask themselves why they are doing this research and what the possible repercussions might be on the participants' lives (Fortin et al., 2009).

Therefore, in nursing research, it is assumed that people's right to privacy is respected and can never be infringed without their consent (International Committee of Medical Journal Editors, 2007). Therefore, no information that allows the identification of the person should be published in the research results and, if identification is essential for scientific purposes, informed consent should be sought. It should be emphasised that confidentiality was ensured at all times during the data collection process for this study.

According to Fortin et al. (2009), any research carried out on human beings raises ethical and moral questions. When individuals are used as subjects in scientific research, great care must be taken to ensure that their rights are protected.

In this sense, the researcher must obtain informed consent in which he or she requests the voluntary participation of the subjects, after having informed them of the objectives of the research and its possible advantages and disadvantages (Fortin, 1999).

Since consent is the agreement given by a person to take part in a study, it must be free and voluntary and the person must fulfil the selected inclusion criteria, being able to change their mind at any time and withdraw from the study if they so wish. For consent to be informed, the person must have all the necessary information to be able to analyse the advantages and disadvantages of taking part (Fortin et al., 2009).

To this end, an informed consent form was drawn up, containing the necessary information to enable people to analyse the advantages and disadvantages of taking part, taking into account the characteristics of the target population and using accessible language, guaranteeing the anonymity and confidentiality of the information collected (Appendix B).

We formally requested authorisation in writing from the author of the questionnaire selected for this study, undertaking to respect the questionnaire, not to make any changes to it and not to publish it (Appendix A).

The Ethics Committee of the respective Local Health Unit (Appendix C) was asked for its opinion, which was positive (Appendix B). The Coordinator of the Outpatient Department and the Head Nurse were informed, and the objectives of the work were communicated, emphasising its interest and importance for improving nursing care for people/families with IBD (Appendix C).

CHAPTER 4

4 - PRESENTATION AND ANALYSIS OF RESULTS

Loyalty Study

The fidelity study of a data collection instrument is an essential component in assessing the accuracy and consistency of the results it provides (Fortin, 2009).

In this study, internal consistency was analysed using the Cronbach's alpha coefficient to estimate the reliability of the scale used and its dimensions (Table 2). Thus, after inverting 3 items (6, 21 and 32), Cronbach's alphas ranging from 0.72 to 0.89 were obtained for the different dimensions of QoL and an alpha of 0.93 for the IBDQ-R as a whole. These values show acceptable internal consistency and are in line with those identified in the study by Veríssimo (2008), which showed a total Cronbach's alpha coefficient of 0.92 and for the different dimensions ranging from 0.77 to 0.87.

Table 2 - Results of the internal consistency using the Cronbach's Alpha coefficient of the IBDQR

	Number of items	a
Intestinal symptoms	10	0,89
Systemic Symptoms	5	0,72
Emotional Aspects	12	0,87
Social aspects	5	0,72
Total IBDQ-R	32	0,93

4.1 - DESCRIPTIVE ANALYSIS

Presentation of results

This part of the paper presents the results obtained according to the methodological strategies used, followed by a discussion of the results, comparing and inferring with similar studies carried out by other authors.

Statistical treatment of data

With regard to analysing the results and in terms of descriptive statistics, the data relating to the demographic and clinical variables and the quality of life of the person with IBD are presented in frequency distribution tables, complemented, whenever the nature of the variable allowed it, by measures of central tendency - mean (M) and median and of dispersion or variability - standard deviation (SD), minimum (Min.) and maximum (Max.).

In order to be able to compare the levels of quality of life between the different dimensions of the IBDQ-R and since each one has a different number of items, it was necessary to calculate the *scores in* two ways:

      a) As recommended by the authors of the scale, that is, by adding up the items that make up each dimension;

      b) By converting to a percentage, i.e. standardising the maximum for each dimension to 100%, which was obtained using the formula: (sum of dimension items*100) /maximum possible dimension score.

The results show both *scores*, which makes it possible to compare the results with those of other studies and also makes it easier to compare, in this sample, the preponderance of each dimension or dimensions for the sample's quality of life.

In terms of inferential analysis, the non-parametric Mann-Whitney U test was used to detect significant differences between the centre values of two groups, the Kruskal-Wallis K test to detect significant differences between the centre values of three or more groups and Spearman's correlation coefficient to assess the correlation between two continuous variables. This choice of non-parametric tests is justified by the small size of the sample, particularly when divided into subgroups to test the hypotheses under study. Although the main dependent variable (QoL) followed a normal distribution ($p>0.05$) for the total sample, verified with the Kolmogorov-Smirnov test with Lilliefors significance correction or, more appropriately, given the size of the sample, by the Shapiro-Wilk test (Table 3), the same is not true when analysing the distribution according to subgroups, such as by gender (Table 4), where it can be seen that the distribution is not normal for men in the "Systemic Symptoms" dimension nor in the total IBDQ-R dimension for women ($p<0,05$).

Chart 3 - Results of the Kolmogorov-Smirnov normality test (with Lilliefors significance correction) and the Shapiro-wilk test for assessing adherence to normality of QoL in people with IBD.

	Kolmogorov-Smirnov with Lilliefors correction	P	Shapiro-Wilk	P
Intestinal symptoms	0,067	0,200	0,978	0,651
Systemic Symptoms	0,161	**0,014**	0,945	0,062
Emotional Aspects	0,069	0,200	0,988	0,941
Social aspects	0,114	0,200	0,965	0,266
Total IBDQ-R	0,114	0,200	0,966	0,298

Table 4 - Results of the application of the Shapiro-Wilk normality test to assess adherence to normality of QoL according to the gender of people with IBD.

Dependent Variable	Gender	Shapiro-Wilk	p
Intestinal symptoms	Female (n=19)	0,976	0,886
	Male (n=19)	0,964	0,658
Systemic Symptoms	Female (n=19)	0,944	0,316
	Male (n=19)	0,885	**0,027**
Emotional Aspects	Female (n=19)	0,958	0,542
	Male (n=19)	0,961	0,587
Social aspects	Female (n=19)	0,931	0,180
	Male (n=19)	0,960	0,574

Total IBDQ-R	Female (n=19)	0,879	**0,021**
	Male (n=19)	0,942	0,291

Because some variables had few observations/counts in some of their categories, they had to be grouped together in order to facilitate the statistical treatment of the data. The following variables were grouped together:

> *Marital status, with* only two categories being considered: **married and unmarried** (including widowers and singles);

> *The level of education,* for two nominal categories of level of education: **lower, up to 9th grade** (encompassing participants with no studies, with fourth grade and 9th grade) and **higher or equal to 12th grade;**

> *Occupation,* for two nominal categories: **employed** or **not employed (the** latter includes the options of unemployed, student or retired);

> **Smoking** *habits,* for two nominal categories: **smokes or has smoked** and has **never smoked**;

> *Alcohol habits,* for two nominal categories: **non-existent habits** and **light or moderate habits**.

A=0.05 was taken as the critical significance value for the results of the hypothesis tests, and the null hypothesis was rejected when the probability of type I error was lower than that value (p<0.05). The IBM® SPSS® version 20 programme was used to statistically process the data.

The results of this study are presented in response to the established objectives and are divided into three main parts:

> characterisation of the sample;

> characterisation of quality of life;

> results of the hypothesis tests.

Characterisation of the sample

A total of 38 people with IBD took part in this study, whose sociodemographic and clinical characteristics are shown in tables 5 and 6. The sample was made up of 19 females (50 per cent) and 19 males (50 per cent), with an average age of 43.20 years (SD±13.50). Most of these people had completed their 12th year of schooling (28.90%) and higher education (28.90%). In terms of marital status, the majority of participants were married (65.80%) and in terms of work activity, the majority were employed (57.80%). In clinical terms, CD was the most representative with 19 people (50.0%), followed by UC with 10 people (26.30%) and undetermined IBD with 9 patients (23.70%). Most people reported never having smoked (65.80%) and not having alcohol habits (71.10%). Fifteen patients (39.50%) were admitted to hospital, the main reasons being haemorrhage (n=4) and worsening of the disease (n=3), while perianal abscesses, early stages of the disease, surgery, diarrhoea, stenosis/surgery, intestinal inflammation, intestinal perforation and side effects to medication were also identified.

Table 5 - Socio-demographic characterisation of the sample

Variables	n	%
Female gender	19	50,00
Male gender	19	50,00
Marital status Single Married Divorced Widowed	11 25 1 1	30,00 65,80 2,60 2,60
Level of education No studies 4.ª Class 9th grade 12th year Higher education	1 8 7 11 11	2,60 21,10 18,40 28,90 28,90
Professional Status Employed Unemployed Student Retired	22 6 5 5	57,80 15,80 13,20 13,20
Pathology Crohn's disease Ulcerative colitis Undetermined IBD	19 10 9	50,00 26,30 23,70
Smoking habits Non-smoker Ex-smoker Smoking	25 9 4	65,80 23,70 10,50
Alcohol habits Non-existent Light Moderate	27 9 2	71,10 23,70 5,30
Hospitalisation	15	39,50

The time since diagnosis ranged from 1 to 29 years, with an average of 8.80 years (SD±7.30).

Chart 6 - Age and time since diagnosis.

	Average	Standard Deviation	Median	Minimum	Maximum
Age (years)	43,20	13,50	43,50	19,00	65,00
Diagnostic time	8,80	7,30	6,00	1,00	29,00

Characterisation of quality of life

An individualised analysis of each item (Table 7) shows that the ones with the highest average, corresponding to the worst situation, were item 11 - "Fear of not finding a toilet nearby" (M=4.10; SD±1.80), item 19 - "Anxiety due to fears related to the illness" (M=3.90; SD±1.60) and item 20 - "Discomfort due to abdominal distension" (M=3.90; SD±1.40). At the opposite end of the spectrum, corresponding to a better situation, was item 22 - "Bleeding when the bowels work" (M=1.90; SD±1.10), item 28 - "Feeling constrained in their sexual activity" (M=2.00; SD±1.10) and item 26 - "Getting their clothes dirty without meaning to" (M=2.20; SD±1.40). Item 21

"Feeling relaxed or at ease" (M=4.00; SD±1.10) was the only one in which no patient recorded the worst possible state, with a minimum value of 2 and one of the highest averages, bearing in mind that this is one of the inverted questions.

Below is the table mentioned above with the results corresponding to the descriptive statistics of the different items (Table 7).

Table 7 - Descriptive statistics for the individual items of the IBDQ-R.

Item*	Average	DP	Median	Min.	Max.
Q1	3,60	1,70	3,00	1	7
Q2	3,50	1,40	4,00	1	6
Q3	3,70	1,40	4,00	1	7
Q4	2,40	1,40	2,00	1	7
Q5	3,30	1,90	4,00	1	7
Q6#	3,70	1,00	4,00	1	5
Q7	3,80	1,90	3,50	1	7
Q8	2,30	1,40	2,00	1	5
Q9	3,60	1,60	4,00	1	7
Q10	3,80	1,40	4,00	1	6
Q11	**4,10**	1,80	4,00	1	7
Q12	3,10	1,50	3,00	1	6
Q13	3,80	1,60	4,00	1	7
Q14	2,80	1,40	2,50	1	6
Q15	3,40	1,50	3,00	1	7
Q16	2,90	1,60	3,00	1	6
Q17	3,10	1,50	3,00	1	6
Q18	3,60	1,60	4,00	1	7
Q19	**3,90**	1,60	4,00	1	7
Q20	**3,90**	1,40	4,00	1	6
Q21#	**4,00**	1,10	4,00	2	7
Q22	_1,90_	1,10	2,00	1	5
Q23	2,40	1,50	2,00	1	6
Q24	3,20	1,50	3,00	1	6
Q25	3,10	1,70	3,00	1	7
Q26	_2,20_	1,40	2,00	1	6
Q27	2,80	1,50	2,50	1	6
Q28	_2,00_	1,10	2,00	1	4
Q29	3,30	1,30	4,00	1	5
Q30	3,80	1,60	4,00	1	7
Q31	2,50	1,70	2,00	1	7
Q32#	3,20	0,90	3,00	1	5

* Each item is measured on a *Likert* scale between 1 and 7 points, with the higher the score the lower the QoL.
ᵉ Item with inverted quotation.

Table 8 shows the average values and variation for each of the dimensions and for the IBDQ-R as a whole. Analysing the normalised values for ease of interpretation, since the results are the same when not normalised, it can be seen that, in average terms, the "Systemic Symptoms" dimension is the one in which the sample shows the highest results (M=49.50, SD±13.40), followed by the "Emotional Aspects" dimension (M=48.40, SD±14.00) and the "Intestinal Symptoms" dimension (M=45.60, SD±15.30), which translates into worse QoL. The dimension in which the sample showed the best QoL was "Social Aspects" (M=36.50, SD±14.00).

It can also be seen that the average of all the QoL dimensions is between 40 and 60, which translates into a reasonable average QoL. Overall, the average score for the IBDQ-R was 45.80 out of 100, with a minimum of 44.00 and a maximum of 72.30.

Table 8 - Descriptive statistics for QoL from the IBDQ-R total by dimension
*The higher the score, the worse the QoL.

	Dimension (possible variation) *	Average	Deviation Standard	Median	Min.	Max.
Sum of the dimensions and Total of the IBDQ-R (32-224)	Intestinal symptoms (10-70)	31,90	10,70	31,50	11,00	52,00
	Systemic symptoms (5-35)	17,30	4,70	18,50	6,00	26,00
	Emotional Aspects (12-84)	40,60	11,80	41,00	16,00	66,00
	Social Aspects (5-35)	12,80	4,90	12,00	5,00	23,00
	Total IBDQ-R (32-224)	102,70	27,50	98,50	42,00	162,00
***Scores* adjusted to 100% of IBDQ-R dimensions and Total**	Intestinal symptoms (0-100)	45,60	15,30	45,00	15,70	74,30
	Systemic Symptoms (0-100)	**49,50**	13,40	52,90	17,10	74,30
	Emotional Aspects (0-100)	48,40	14,00	48,80	19,00	78,60
	Social Aspects (0-100)	**36,50**	14,00	34,30	14,30	65,70
	Total IBDQ-R (0-100)	45,80	12,30	44,00	1,80	72,30

4.2 - INFERENTIAL ANALYSIS

Hypothesis testing

We will now present the results of the statistical tests carried out to test the hypotheses.

Hypothesis 1 - There is a relationship between the perception of the QoL of people with IBD and sociodemographic variables;

H1.1 - The perception of the QoL of people with IBD is influenced by Gender

The Mann-Whitney *U-test was* used to compare QoL between men and women (Table 9), and there were no statistically significant differences for any of the dimensions or for the total IBDQ-R (p>0.05). There is therefore no evidence to say that the perception of QoL is influenced by being a man or a woman with IBD.

Chart 9 - Comparison of the perception of the QoL of people with IBD according to gender.

	Gender	n	Average posts	Median	U	p
Intestinal symptoms (10-70)	Female	19	23,00	36,00	114,00	0,053
	Male	19	16,00	30,00		
Systemic Symptoms (5-35)	Female	19	22,90	19,00	116,00	0,061
	Male	19	16,10	18,00		
Emotional Aspects (12-84)	Female	19	22,90	42,00	115,50	0,057
	Male	19	16,10	38,00		
Social Aspects (5-35)	Female	19	20,70	12,00	158,00	0,525
	Male	19	18,30	13,00		
Total IBDQ-R (32-224)	Female	19	22,50	112,00	124,00	0,103
	Male	19	16,50	98,00		

H1.2 - The perception of QoL of people with IBD is influenced by marital status

Since there was only one divorced and one widowed person, they were grouped together as unmarried (along with the single people) and compared to the married (Table 10). There was no statistically significant difference in QoL between these two categories, i.e. there is no statistical evidence to say that marital status (married versus unmarried) influences the perception that people with IBD have of their QoL.

Chart 10 - Comparison of the perception of the QoL of people with IBD according to marital status.

	Marital status	n	Average posts	Median	U	p
Intestinal symptoms (10-70)	**Married**	25	17,70	30,00	116,50	0,159
	Not married	13	23,00	36,00		
Systemic symptoms (5-35)	**Married**	25	18,50	18,00	137,50	0,447
	Not married	13	21,40	19,00		
Emotional Aspects (12-84)	**Married**	25	18,70	40,00	141,50	0,523
	Not married	13	21,10	43,00		
Social Aspects (5-35)	**Married**	25	18,70	11,00	143,50	0,564
	Not married	13	21,00	13,00		
Total IBDQ-R (32-224)	**Married**	25	17,90	98.0	121,50	0,210
	Not married	13	22,70	112.00		

H1.3 - The perception of the QoL of people with IBD is influenced by the level of education.

In order to assess the influence of level of education on QoL, the sample was divided into two groups, those below and above the 12th year of schooling (Table 11). A statistically significant difference was only found for the "Social Aspects" dimension (p<0.05), with QoL in this area being higher in people with a higher level of schooling (median of 15.50 versus 11.00). Thus, given the results obtained, it can be said that the higher the level of schooling, the more evidence there is that people have a better perception of their QoL in the "Social Aspects" dimension.

Chart 11 - Comparison of the perception of the QoL of people with IBD according to their level of education.

	Level of education	n	Average posts	Median	U	p
Intestinal symptoms (10-70)	Up to 9th grade	16	17,20	28,50	213,50	0,271
	12th grade or higher	22	21,20	35,00		
Systemic symptoms (5-35)	Up to 9th grade	16	19,60	18,00	174,50	0,965
	12th grade or higher	22	19,40	19,00		
Emotional Aspects (12-84)	Up to 9th grade	16	20,20	40,50	165.5	0,759
	12th grade or higher	22	19,00	41,50		
Social Aspects (5-35)	Up to 9th grade	16	24,40	15,50	97.5	**0,020**
	12th grade or higher	22	15,90	11,00		
Total IBDQ-R (32-224)	Up to 9th grade	16	20,30	103,00	163.5	0,711
	12th grade or higher	22	18,90	98,00		

H1.4 -The perceived QoL of people with IBD is influenced by their professional situation

In order to assess the influence of professional status on the perception of QoL, the sample was also grouped into two groups, employed and non-employed, the latter category including the unemployed, students and pensioners (Table 12). There was no statistically significant difference, so there is no statistical evidence to say that professional status influences the perceived QoL of IBD patients.

Chart 12 - Comparison of the perception of the QoL of people with IBD according to their professional situation.

	Professional Status	n	Average posts	Median	U	p
Intestinal symptoms (10-70)	Employee	22	22,00	35,00	122,00	0,110
	Not employed	16	16,10	29,50		
Systemic symptoms (5-35)	Employee	22	19,80	19,00	169,00	0,849
	Not employed	16	19,10	18,00		
Emotional Aspects (12-84)	Employee	22	20,80	42,00	147,50	0,404
	Not employed	16	17,70	38,00		
Social Aspects (5-35)	Employee	22	17,80	11,00	213,00	0,284
	Not employed	16	21,80	13,50		
Total IBDQ-R (32-224)	Employee	22	20,20	98,50	160,00	0,651
	Not employed	16	18,50	100,50		

Hypothesis 2 - There is a relationship between the perception of the QoL of people with IBD and behavioural habits;

H 2.1 - The perceived QoL of people with IBD is influenced by smoking habits

Comparing the QoL of people with IBD who smoke or have ever smoked with people who have never smoked (Table 13), there is a statistically significant difference in the "Social Aspects" dimension and in the total IBDQ-R, with those who smoke or have ever smoked having a better QoL in social terms (median of 10.00 versus 14.00) and in the total scale (median of 89.00 versus 105.00).

Chart 13 - Comparison of the perception of the QoL of people with IBD according to the existence of smoking habits.

	Smoking	n	Average posts	Median	U	p
Intestinal symptoms (10-70)	Smokes or has smoked	13	14,70	28.00	100,50	0,056
	Never smoked	25	22,00	35.00		
Systemic Symptoms (5-35)	Smokes or has smoked	13	16,30	17,00	121,00	0,199
	Never smoked	25	21,20	19,00		
Emotional Aspects (12-84)	Smokes or has smoked	13	17,80	40,00	140,00	0,488
	Never smoked	25	20,40	41,00		
Social Aspects (5-35)	Smokes or has smoked	13	14,10	10,00	92,00	**0,030**
	Never smoked	25	22,30	14,00		
Total IBDQ-R (32-224)	Smokes or has smoked	13	14,10	89,00	92,00	**0,030**
	Never smoked	25	22,30	105,00		

H 2.2 -The perceived QoL of people with IBD is influenced by the existence of alcohol habits

When comparing the perceived QoL of people with mild or moderate alcohol habits with those with no alcohol habits (Table 14), there were no statistically significant differences between the two groups (p>0.05).

Chart 14 - Comparison of the perception of the QoL of people with IBD according to the existence of alcohol habits.

	Alcohol habits	n	Average posts	Median	U	p
Intestinal symptoms (10-70)	Nonexistent	27	21,10	35,00	104.50	0,156
	Mild or moderate	11	15,50	29,00		
Systemic Symptoms (5-35)	Nonexistent	27	21,50	19,00	93,50	0,075
	Mild or moderate	11	14,50	18,00		

Emotional Aspects (12-84)	Nonexistent	27	21,00	42,00	108,50	0,198
	Mild or moderate	11	15,90	38,00		
Social Aspects (5-35)	Nonexistent	27	20,30	12,00	127,00	0,487
	Mild or moderate	11	17,60	11,00		
Total IBDQ- R (32-224)	Nonexistent	27	21,10	103,00	105,00	0,161
	Mild or moderate	11	15,60	91,00		

Hypothesis 3 - There is a relationship between the perception of the QoL of people with IBD and clinical variables

H 3.1 - The perception of the QoL of people with IBD is influenced by the confirmation of the diagnosis

The perception of QoL was compared between people with CD, UC and undetermined IBD (Table 15), and there were no statistically significant differences in the perception of QoL between the three groups.

Chart 15 - Comparison of the perception of QoL of people with IBD according to the type of pathology.

	Pathology	n	Median	K	P
Intestinal symptoms (10-70)	Crohn's disease	19	30,00	3,392	0,183
	Ulcerative colitis	10	36,50		
	Undetermined IBD	9	30,00		
Systemic Symptoms (5-35)	Crohn's disease	19	19,00	1,025	0,599
	Ulcerative colitis	10	17,50		
	Undetermined IBD	9	17,00		
Emotional Aspects (12-84)	Crohn's disease	19	40,00	4,078	0,130
	Ulcerative colitis	10	44,00		
	Undetermined IBD	9	31,00		
Social Aspects (5-35)	Crohn's disease	19	13,00	3,352	0,187
	Ulcerative colitis	10	14,50		
	Undetermined IBD	9	11,00		
Total IBDQ-R (32-224)	Crohn's disease	19	98,00	3,592	0,166
	Ulcerative colitis	10	110,00		
	Undetermined IBD	9	87,00		

H 3.2 - The perception of the QoL of people with IBD is influenced by the need for hospitalisation

Comparing the perception of QoL between people who were and were not hospitalised (Table 16), it was found that the former had better QoL in terms of the "Social Aspects" dimension (median of 16.00 versus 11.00), with no statistically significant differences in the other dimensions or in the total *score.*

Chart 16 - Comparison of the perception of the QoL of people with IBD according to whether they were hospitalised.

	Hospitalisation	n	Average posts	Median	U	p
Intestinal symptoms (10-70)	No	23	18,70	32,00	190,50	0,591
	Yes	15	20,70	30,00		
Systemic Symptoms (5-35)	No	23	19,80	19,00	165,00	0,822
	Yes	15	19,00	18,00		
Emotional Aspects (12-84)	No	23	17,50	38,00	217,50	0,179
	Yes	15	22,50	42,00		
Social Aspects (5-35)	No	23	16,20	11,00	248,50	**0,022**
	Yes	15	24,60	16,00		
Total IBDQ-R (32-224)	No	23	17,87	98,00	210,00	0,273
	Yes	15	22,00	116,00		

H 3.3 -The perceived QoL of people with IBD is influenced by the time of diagnosis

The correlation between the number of years since diagnosis and the perception of QoL in people with IBD was tested (Table 17) and no statistically significant correlation was found (p>0.05).

Chart 17 - Correlation between time since diagnosis (years) and perception of QoL in people with IBD.

	Years of diagnosis	
	lol	P
Intestinal symptoms	0,039	0,817
Systemic Symptoms	0,081	0,628
Emotional Aspects	0,070	0,678
Social aspects	0,005	0,978
Total IBDQ-R	0,023	0,890

5 - DISCUSSION OF RESULTS

Interpreting quality of life is not easy, because the idea is complex, ambiguous and differs according to culture, time and person, and changes over time and circumstances. The idea of QoL and well-being has varied over time and is increasingly valued these days.

The concept of QoL is defined by a person's subjective assessment of their physical and mental health and social status, taking into account their own experiences of health and illness (Neubauer, Arlukiewicz and Paradowski, 2009).

For Sampaio (2007), quality of life reflects the degree of awareness that each person has in relation to real life and individual expectations, thus reflecting the person's own goals and dreams.

With the aim of finding out the perception of the quality of life of people with inflammatory bowel disease enrolled in the Outpatient Clinic of a Local Health Unit in the Centre Region, a sample of 38 participants was obtained, which was evenly distributed in terms of gender, consisting of 19 men and 19 women. The average age of the participants was 43.20 years, with a minimum of 19 years and a maximum of 65 years. The time since diagnosis varied between 1 and 29 years, with an average of 8.80 years (SD±7.30).

In this context, there is a predominance of a young population, similar to other studies such as Souza et al. (2008), where the distribution of IBD in Brazilian patients is higher in the age group between 20 and 39 years with an average age of 37.50 years and in the study by Souza, Barbosa, Espinosa and Belasco (2011) which shows a greater distribution of IBD in the age group between 20 and 41 years, with an average age of 40.20 years. The study by Silva (2015) also shows that the age of people with IBD is between 20 and 40.

In line with this data, the study carried out by Saurabh and Ahuja (2017) in the Indian population concludes that IBD affects young and active people and is associated with significant losses in functional capacity and autonomy.

In the Portuguese study by Trindade et al. (2016), in which 200 IBD patients took part, it was found that the majority were women, with an average age of 35.85 years, which is not in line with the data obtained in this study, since no gender differences were identified and the average age was higher at 42.30 years.

In the study carried out by Souza et al. (2011), there was also a greater predominance of females (62.00%).

Alowais, Alferayan and Aljehani (2016) carried out a study on the QoL of people with IBD involving 32 participants, 20 of whom were male and 12 female, which is not very consistent with the other studies carried out in this field, in that it is the female gender that is most affected. The average age was 34.28 years, which reflects the general tendency for the young population to be affected.

Magalhães et al. (2015) carried out a study with a sample of 85 patients, 64.40 per cent of whom were female and with an average age of 39.30 years, which is lower than the present study.

CD was the most representative in this study, with a total of 19 patients (50.00%), followed by ulcerative colitis with 10 patients (26.30%) and finally undetermined IBD with 9 patients (23.70%).

Regarding the distribution of the disease, there are several studies that are in agreement with the present one, such as the one by Coelho (2010) in which, in a sample of 58 participants, 31 people had CD and 27 had UC; the one by Ramos, Calvet, Sicilia et al. (2015), in which 293 people took part, 151 had CD and 142 had UC; Magalhães et al. (2015), with a sample of 85 participants in which 55 had CD and 30 had UC; and Juillerat, Pittet, Bulliard et al. (2008), with 1,016 participants, with a higher number of cases of CD compared to UC, although not significantly.

In the study by Alowais, Alferayan and Aljehani (2016), of the 32 participants, 16 had CD and 16 had UC. Torres et al. (2011), with 103 participants, obtained results of 62 with UC and 41 with CD, and Souza et al. (2011) with 49 participants, 18 had CD (36.70%) and 31 UC (63.20%), making it clear that the largest number of participants suffered from UC, which is not in line with the data obtained in the present study.

According to Neubauer, et al. (2009), patients with CD mostly live alone and do not form a family in the sense of having children, and they are at greater risk of absenteeism from work with the need to resort to support from allowances or sickness benefits.

The majority of the participants in this study were married (65.80%), had a 12th grade education (28.90%) and higher education (28.90%), and the majority were employed (57.80%).

In the study carried out by Coelho (2010), the majority of participants were married (65.50 per cent), although there was a higher percentage of people with a level of education corresponding to the 9th year of schooling (56.90 per cent) and a higher percentage of unemployed people (55.10 per cent), contrary to this study.

Souza et al. (2011), in their study, show the same trend in terms of marital status, with a higher number of married people (69.90 per cent).

In the study by Ramos, Calvet, Sicilia et al. (2015), the majority were employed as in the present study.

The pathogenesis of IBD is not yet fully understood; however, it is known that both genetic and environmental factors (smoking, intestinal bacterial flora and appendectomy) can play a fundamental role in deregulating the intestinal immune balance, leading to the development of lesions (Pereira, 2014).

The relationship between smoking habits and IBD has been recognised for some years, and tobacco consumption is considered one of the most important environmental factors in the pathogenesis of chronic IBD. The numerous existing epidemiological studies that describe this relationship still know little about the molecular and cellular mechanisms triggered in the intestine by the influence of tobacco, which could lead, under certain circumstances, to the development of CD or the prevention of UC (Pereira, 2014).

In this study, the majority of participants reported never having smoked (65.80%) and not having alcohol habits (71.10%), which is in line with the study carried out by Coelho (2010) in which they reported 54 non-smokers (93.10%) and 4 smokers (6.90%). In the study by Souza et al. (2011), 51 participants were smokers (49.50%) and 52 non-smokers (50.50%), and the difference between the two was not significant.

After analysing the data from this study, we can conclude that 15 people (39.50%) were hospitalised due to various complications, most notably haemorrhage (n=4); exacerbation of the disease (n=3) and stenosis/surgery (n=2).

In the study by Coelho (2010), intestinal surgery was performed on 6 people, 5 with CD (16.10%) and 1 with UC (3.70%), and 5 people with CD were hospitalised (8.62%). In the study by Magalhães et al. (2015), with 85 participants, 27 had CD and underwent surgery (31.80%) and 7 people had a history of perianal disease (8.20%). 47 people (55.30%) had already been hospitalised for IBD, 40 of whom had CD and 7 had UC.

IBD has been increasing in incidence, affecting young people. In this sense, the QoL of these people has been explored on an ongoing basis because, given the characteristics of this disease, which involve the need for several episodes of hospitalisation and surgical interventions, it is understandable that this has a direct impact on their well-being (Raposo, 2008). Despite these implications, it is known that medical and surgical developments have increased life expectancy, and it is essential to understand what affects the quality of life of these people in order to act to minimise the negative effects and enhance the positive aspects.

People with IBD in remission have altered levels of QoL compared to normally healthy people (Trindade et al., 2016). This study found that the average of all the QoL dimensions was below 50.00% (between 40 and 60%), which translates into a reasonable average QoL. On average, the "Systemic Symptoms", "Emotional Aspects" and "Intestinal Symptoms" dimensions show higher results, which translates into worse QoL, while the dimension in which the sample showed the best QoL was the "Social Aspects" dimension. The results obtained in this study are not in agreement with those obtained in the study by Coelho (2010) which used the same instrument, but with reformulated questions and inverted scoring, which revealed that the dimension with the worst results in terms of QoL was the "Systemic Symptoms" dimension and the one with the best results was the "Emotional Aspects" dimension. The study by Trindade et al. (2016) on the QoL of people with IBD, using other measuring instruments, states that all domains of QoL (physical, psychological, social and environmental) show a negative relationship with IBD symptoms, with direct implications for the psychological well-being and QoL of people with IBD, showing a higher incidence during the active phase of the disease compared to the remission phase.

According to the application of the IBDQ-R in the study by Alowais et al. (2016), people reported a low level of QoL, with the dimensions "Social Aspects" and "Systemic Symptoms" having more impact than the dimensions "Emotional Aspects" and "Intestinal Symptoms", which is not in agreement with the present study. Cohen, Bin and Fayh (2010) found that the dimensions with the greatest impact on QoL were "Emotional Aspects" and "Systemic Symptoms", which is in line with the literature and the present study, arguing for the negative impact of emotional and systemic aspects on the QoL of these people, and it can be concluded that the disease in its active phase has a negative influence on all the dimensions of these people's QoL.

The physical domain of QoL is affected by symptoms and the occurrence of complications associated with IBD, which can lead to pain and negative thoughts that condition a person's psychological and social experience.
patient. In this sense, Trindade et al. (2016) conclude that people with IBD in Portugal have lower levels of QoL than the general population in all domains, but with greater visibility in the physical domain and in the total of the instrument they used.

According to the aforementioned authors, the effects of intestinal symptoms on people's lives are most evident in the active phase of the disease, with consequent implications for their ability to fulfil their activities of daily living, work and leisure. Magalhães et al. (2015) are of the same opinion, stating that IBD causes changes at a physical, psychological and social level, which has a strong impact on people's ability to carry out their activities of daily living autonomously and without limitations, as it is characterised by frequent hospitalisations and prolonged treatments.

When each item was analysed, the items with the worst scores were "Fear of not finding a toilet nearby" (M=4.10), "Anxiety due to fears related to the disease" (M=3.90) and "Discomfort due to abdominal distension" (M=3.90), which will have a negative influence on these people's QoL, which is understandable given the symptoms and complications of the disease. In the study carried out by Coelho (2010), the items that influenced a lower QoL were "Fear of not finding a toilet nearby", as in the present study, "Having gas", "Fatigue/tiredness" and "Difficulties in leisure/sports activities".

People's concerns centre on their weakness, their difficulty in maintaining their activities of daily living and their fear of the prognosis and the future (Trindade et al.,

2016). The fear of the disease developing into a neoplasm is a constant concern for people/families with IBD, since they are known to be at high risk of developing this pathology, and surveillance and screening programmes should be implemented in order to make an early diagnosis (Raposo, 2008).

On the other hand, the items with the lowest scores that correspond to a better QoL are "Bleeding with bowel movements" (M=1.90), "Feeling constrained in their sexual activity" (M=2.00) and "Getting their clothes dirty without wanting to" (M=2.20), which is in line with the study by Coelho (2010), who showed similar results for the last two items mentioned.

The importance of an active sexuality has a direct influence on the ability to have and maintain a healthy intimate relationship, without fear or pain. A large majority of people with IBD are young, of reproductive age and, as such, are worried about rejection and lack of sexual interest related to all the manifestations of the disease (Barros, 2016).

Despite being a controversial and complex subject, and due to the scarcity of scientific studies in this field, Barros (2016) considered it appropriate to study the consequences of IBD on people's sexuality, having defined the objective of the study as assessing the prevalence of sexual dysfunction in people with IBD and identifying the clinical and psychological factors associated with it. Contrary to this study, it concluded that sexual dysfunction is frequent in people with IBD, especially in women. The factors associated with erectile dysfunction in men were weight loss, fatigue, weakness, perianal surgery in people with CD, the presence of perianal disease, depression, low self-esteem and worse QoL. The factors associated with sexual dysfunction in women were dyspareunia and lack of vaginal lubrication.

Although sexual changes are common in chronic illness, people don't talk openly about this subject, because sexuality is still surrounded by prejudices and taboos and, as a result, people have little information and show fear and inhibition in seeking it out. The use of specific scales and questionnaires can facilitate an initial approach, allowing the person to recognise their problem and start a more natural dialogue with the nursing and medical team or a psychologist (Barros, 2016).

Interpersonal relationships, sexual and emotional intimacy, self-image and sexual activity are topics that should be addressed with everyone, including those suffering from IBD. Working as part of a multidisciplinary team is essential, as it is this interprofessional relationship that will enable greater attention to be paid to the questions, doubts and anxieties faced by the person and their family. In this context, it is imperative that people's needs are taken into account, including emotional and sexual aspects related to IBD and the impact it has on their personal and family life (Barros, 2016).

With regard to the item "Feeling relaxed or at ease", it can be seen that this was the only one in which no patient recorded the worst possible state, with a minimum value of 2 and one of the highest averages (M=4.00), bearing in mind that this is one of the inverted items, which translates into better QoL.

Moving on to the discussion of the *inferential statistics* carried out and with regard to the relationship between the sociodemographic characterisation and the QoL of people with IBD, it was found that there is no statistical evidence to affirm that the gender of people with IBD has an influence on their QoL levels.

There are studies that show that women are at greater risk of having lower levels of QoL, as they are more concerned about their state of health and issues related to self-image (Neubauer, et al., 2009; Magalhães et al., 2015). In contrast, Souza et al. (2011) in their study show that there is a higher prevalence in females, with significantly better levels of QoL compared to males.

Regarding the influence of marital status on the QoL of people with IBD, there were no statistically significant differences, i.e. there is no statistical evidence to say that marital status influences the QoL of people with IBD. This finding is in line with most of the studies analysed (Neubauer, et al., 2009).

The level of education has been shown to be important in some studies, as it has been proven that the higher the level, the better the quality of life of people with IBD (Casellas, Lopez-Vivancos, Casado and Malagelada, 2002; Coelho, 2010). The same trend can be seen in the present sample, as there is a statistically significant difference in the "Social Aspects" dimension, with QoL in this area being higher in people with a higher level of education.

This may be related to the fact that people with training have access to more information and are better able to internalise IBD-related content, which leads to a better understanding of the disease and therefore a more effective way of developing strategies to reduce anxiety levels.

With regard to the relationship between the professional situation and the QoL of people with IBD, there was no statistically significant difference, and there is no statistical evidence to say that being employed or not can influence the quality of life of people with IBD.

According to Magalhães, et al. (2015), the difficulties faced by people with IBD are reflected in economic and social terms, since 20 per cent of the participants receive a benefit or disability pension and 10 to 25 per cent are at risk of unemployment. In the study by Ramos et al. (2015), out of a total of 293 participants with IBD, 214 were workers, 12 were receiving a disability pension, 16 were unemployed and 11 were in the process of losing their jobs due to recurrent absenteeism from work.

Analysing the results of these studies, it can be seen that people with IBD are very likely to have their professional lives altered due to the exacerbation of the symptoms of the disease, which can lead to absenteeism from work, the need for hospitalisation or, in a more complicated phase, the interruption of professional activity. In this study, of the 38 participants, 16 were unemployed, including students, the unemployed and pensioners, and the difference between the employed and the unemployed was not significant, with a difference of 6 participants.

In the relationship between behavioural habits, which analysed the existence of smoking and alcohol habits and the QoL of people with IBD, there was a statistically significant difference in the "Social Aspects" dimension and in the total *score, with* those who smoke or have smoked having a better QoL in the "Social Aspects" dimension. There were no statistically significant differences between people with mild or moderate alcohol habits and those with no alcohol habits in terms of their influence on QoL.

The aetiological causes of IBD have not yet been identified, but factors such as smoking habits and appendectomy are thought to have a strong influence (Loftus, 2004). Several studies have concluded that smokers have a lower quality of life and that smoking habits favour the development of IBD, especially UC (Raposo, 2008; Souza et al., 2011). In the analysis carried out in his study, Santos (2015) considers that tobacco consumption is a risk factor for CD, although, paradoxically, it seems to be a protective factor for UC. In the study carried out by Pereira (2014), it was concluded that in general, tobacco appears to have a favourable effect on the colon, although in the small intestine it appears to be more harmful, demonstrating a potential increase in susceptibility to the development of an inflammatory process.

Tobacco appears to be less harmful to the colon than to the ileum, and it is the localisation of the disease that determines the effect and involvement of tobacco in the development of IBD. Bearing in mind the conclusions of these studies, the establishment of a causal relationship between smoking and the development of IBD and, consequently, its impact on the QoL of these people is not scientifically rigorous.

In this study, as mentioned above, there is a statistically significant relationship between the existence of smoking habits and the quality of life of people with IBD in the "Social Aspects" dimension and in the total scale, with those who smoke or have smoked having better levels of QoL.

Regarding the relationship between alcohol habits and the QoL of life of people with IBD, the literature search showed that there is no scientific evidence in this area. However, and taking this reality into account, Santos (2015) states in his study that, although there are still no enlightening studies on the factors that interfere with IBD, some attention has been paid to the effect of an inadequate diet, alcohol consumption, *stress,* sleep disorders, exposure to antibiotics, antivirals and bacterial infections on the QoL of people with IBD.

With regard to the relationship between the type of disease (CD or UC) and the QoL of people with IBD, there were no statistically significant differences. There was also no statistically significant correlation between QoL and years since diagnosis. The study carried out by Cohen et al. (2010) is in line with the results obtained in the present study, in that it found that the QoL of people with IBD does not differ in relation to the presence of CD or UC, as long as they are in remission, and it is the state of disease activity that proves to be a preponderant factor influencing the level of QoL.

Coelho (2010) and Alowais et al. (2016) concluded in their studies on the QoL of people with IBD that people with CD have worse levels of QoL.

The clinical manifestation of IBD is varied and depends on the activity and type of the disease. The quality of life of a person with CD is lower, not only when compared to the healthy population, but also when compared to people with UC. The study by Neubauer et al. (2009) found that the factor that most influenced QoL was the activity of the disease, regardless of the duration of the disease, since this was the aspect that most affected people with a diagnosis of less than 5 years, while for those with a diagnosis of between 5 and 9 years, it was the length of hospitalisation that had the greatest influence on QoL. Physical disability is frequent and worsens over time, since after 10 years of diagnosis, approximately 50% of people had some kind of recognised disability (Ramos et al., 2015).

For Dur, Sadlonova, Haider et al. (2014), in their study on the determinants of well-being and QoL in people with CD, the time since diagnosis of the disease was longer in women, although they were younger than men and had lower levels of QoL. These results may be related to the fact that, over the course of the diagnosed disease, men are able to develop more *coping* strategies and thus demonstrate a greater capacity for resilience.

In the literature consulted, it was found that disease activity is the most worrying variable for younger people with fewer years of illness, as they tend to overvalue the symptoms, making them their focus of attention. More experienced sufferers are more concerned about absenteeism from work, the need for hospitalisation or the effects of long-term corticosteroid use (Magalhães et al., 2015).

When comparing QoL between people who have been hospitalised and those who have not, this study found that the former have better QoL in terms of "Social Aspects", with no statistically significant differences in the other dimensions or in the total scale.

IBD affects young people into adulthood, interfering with every aspect of their lives. Around half of people suffer frequent relapses or have ongoing disease activity. Around two-thirds of people with CD still develop complications that require multiple hospitalisations and surgical interventions, yet some recent studies suggest that surgical interventions have decreased in UC and CD (Raposo, 2008; Burisch, et al., 2013). In this context, the risk of imminent psychological changes is understandable, with a consequent reduction in QoL levels (Raposo, 2008).

As mentioned above, CD and UC require numerous hospitalisations and lengthy treatments, which has direct implications for the well-being of these people, affecting various areas of life, namely the physical, mental and social, which consequently have a strong impact on people's ability to carry out their activities of daily living autonomously and without limitations. In the study carried out by the European Federation of Crohn's & Ulcerative Colitis Associations in conjunction with the European Crohn's and Colitis Organisation (2013), it was found that more than half of those surveyed feel that their quality of life is affected by IBD, with 26% needing to stop working for more than 25 days a year, having to resort to sickness benefits to meet their financial needs, and around a quarter of them even losing their jobs (Magalhães et al., 2015). The study by Coelho (2010) concluded that people who had been hospitalised had lower IBDQ-R scores, with a more significant impact on the "Systemic Symptoms" and "Social Aspects" domains.

The subject of the Quality of Life of people with Inflammatory Bowel Disease is pertinent and challenging, and should be developed in order to obtain results that will add value to their improvement.

CHAPTER 6

CONCLUSION

Research is an extremely important area for nursing and for the quality of care provided in the context of disease prevention and health promotion, with direct visibility on the quality of life of people in general and those with inflammatory bowel disease in particular.

Crohn's Disease and Ulcerative Colitis are two chronic IBDs of unknown etiology, characterised by periods of exacerbation alternating with periods of remission. They are associated with significant morbidity, requiring a variety of treatments that can culminate in surgical intestinal resection. The predominance of these pathologies is more evident in the working population, with symptoms that are, in most cases, incapacitating for work and strongly detrimental to people's quality of life, requiring specific measures to be taken to control symptoms in order to minimise their effects (Order No. 9767/2014).

The term health-related quality of life is essential for humanity and for evaluating the effectiveness of health services, because factors such as psychological well-being or malaise seem to have an influence on the functioning of the organism and the evolution of the disease, on the effect of therapy and even on longevity itself, and one of the main objectives of health care is to increase people's QoL (Pinto and Ribeiro, 2006).

It is not the absolute ambition of this study to make an exhaustive assessment of the QoL of people with IBD, as we know how difficult it is to clarify and study, given its subjectivity. In this sense, its ambition is to try to assess some factors that could be accepted as influencing the perception of QoL of these people, namely those enrolled in a Local Health Unit in the Centre Region.

The study sample consisted of 38 participants with IBD, with an average age of 43.20 years and an even distribution in terms of gender. The majority were married (65.80%), had a level of education higher than or equal to the 12th grade (57.80%), and in terms of labour activity, the majority were employed (57.80%). CD was the most representative with a total of 19 patients (50.00%), followed by UC with 10 patients (26.30%) and, finally, undetermined IBD with 9 patients (23.70%).

The results of the study show that these people consider their perception of QoL to be reasonable (45.80 per cent), which came as a surprise to the researcher given that we know the impact of this disease on the way people experience life in the different dimensions that make it up, knowing that the symptoms of the disease lead to changes in attitudes and behaviour, as well as in physical, social and emotional aspects, with greater evidence during periods of exacerbation.

Most of the sociodemographic and clinical factors were not determinants of QoL, but the occurrence of hospitalisation, evidence of smoking habits or level of education did influence the participants' perception of QoL.

Analysing each item on the scale used, it was found that the items that had a negative influence on QoL were "Fear of not finding a toilet nearby", "Anxiety due to fears related to the illness" and "Discomfort due to abdominal distension". On the other hand, the items that corresponded to a better QoL were "Bleeding during bowel movements", "Feeling restricted in their sexual activity" and "Getting their clothes dirty without meaning to", as these were aspects that happened less frequently in the last fortnight prior to filling in the scale.

Given the impact that IBD has on people's perception of their QoL, its assessment is extremely important. Identifying symptomatic factors or the role that social and emotional factors play in the development of the pathology allows for a subjective assessment of the knowledge of health status. In the long term, evaluating the perception of QoL in health practice can help health professionals understand the health condition of each patient and thus develop strategies to solve the problem.

In this sense, and according to Regulation 128/201, published in the Official Gazette on 18 February 2011, the Community and Public Health Nursing Specialist has a set of knowledge, skills and abilities that they mobilise in the context of clinical practice, enabling them to assess the health needs of the target group and act in all contexts of people's lives, at different levels of prevention. Their work is therefore aimed at the health projects of groups experiencing health/disease processes, community and environmental processes, with a view to health promotion, disease prevention and treatment, functional readaptation and social reintegration in all aspects of life. In the community, the Nurse Specialising in Community Nursing has a key role to play, as they have a broader field of intervention, not only looking at the sick person as the target of intervention, but also their family and surroundings (OE, 2011e).

This work has ensured a deeper understanding of the issue. As well as personal enrichment, it will also raise public awareness of a problem that is becoming increasingly significant.

It is considered to have been a stimulating and very rewarding experience for the author's personal, professional and academic development. The role of the Nurse Specialising in Community Nursing must be highlighted and, as such, can make an essential contribution to providing quality care and promoting health, with the aim of improving the quality of life of people with IBD.

We therefore hope to contribute, albeit in a small way, to awakening people and health professionals, particularly Community Nursing Specialists, to an understanding of the impact of IBD on people, seeking to develop strategies for providing global and holistic care that is appropriate to each person's experience and favourable to an effective process of recovery and acceptance of their condition as "chronically ill", with a view to improving the quality of care provided and achieving health gains for people with this pathology.

Limitations of the study

Drawing up a research study involves outlining specific strategies and objectives that guide the researcher to fulfil all the required methodological principles.

Throughout the process of preparing this study, the author was faced with some logistical and time constraints, namely the difficulties inherent in the data collection process, since after the ethics committee and the institution's Board of Directors had given a positive opinion and authorised the use of the questionnaires, the respective consultation was suspended due to a lack of a speciality doctor, and a convenience sample of people with IBD who had attended other speciality consultations related to the pathology in question had to be used.

In this sense, the sample size was reduced and the data collection period was extended as far as possible, in line with the time required by the School of Health to complete this cycle of studies. As a result, the inference of conclusions and effective results was more limited, and it was not possible to extrapolate to the population that met the study criteria in an objective and linear way.

Suggestions for future studies

In terms of data collection, we suggest selecting an institution where the speciality consultation is in operation, in order to facilitate obtaining a larger and more representative sample of the specificities of this population. The ideal would be to have a wider sample, including other hospitals in order to carry out a more comprehensive study, to enable a better understanding of the reality of the disease, providing better health and social support for people with IBD.

For future work, we suggest including a validated instrument that studies people's well-being, in order to relate this variable to the others included in the study.

One of the aims of carrying out studies in this area would be to create a nursing consultation to provide more appropriate support for people with IBD. This would promote greater involvement by nursing professionals in mobilising teaching and support strategies, providing these people and their families with a private space to express their fears, anxieties and doubts. This action would involve the entire multi-professional team in order to support these people on a psychological and physical level, in order to educate and promote better adaptation/acceptance of their health condition and their training in decision-making, problem-solving and critical thinking, in order to make the right choices about their behaviours in a salutogenic way.

BIBLIOGRAPHICAL REFERENCES

Central Administration of the Health System (2009). *Gastroenterology Hospital Referral Network*. Lisbon: 64 p. ISBN 9789899622609. Accessed on September

03, 2017 at: http://www2.acss.min-saude.pt/Portals/0/Gastrenterologia.pdf.

Alowais, F. A., Alferayan, Y. A. and Aljehani, R. M. (2016). Inflammatory Bowel Disease and Quality of Life in King Abdulaziz Medical City. *Open journal of Gastroenterology*, 6, 11-16.

Anes, E. J. and Ferreira, P. L. (2009). Quality of life in dialysis. *Portuguese Journal of Public Health,* 8, 67-82.

Azevedo, L.F., Magro, F., Portela, F., Lago, P., Deus, J., Cotter, J. et al (2010). Estimating the prevalence of inflammatory bowel disease in Portugal using a pharmaco-epidemiological approach. *Pharmacoepidemiology and drug safety.* Accessed on September 03, 2017, at:
file:///C:/Users/user/Desktop/dissertação%20mestrado/bibliografia%20da%20tese/DII/azevedo_2010.pdf.

Backes, D. S., Backes, M. S., Erdmann, A. L. and Buscher, A. (2012). The professional role of nurses in the Unified Health System: from community health to the family health strategy. *Ciência & Saúde Coletiva,* 17(1), 223-230. Accessed on September 10, 2017, at:
http://www.scielo.br/pdf/csc/v17n1/a24v17n1.pdf.

Barros, J. R. (2016). *Sexuality and inflammatory bowel diseases.* Thesis for a Master's degree in Pathophysiology in Clinical Medicine. Universidade Estadual Paulista "Júlio de Mesquita Filho", Botucatu Campus. Accessed on 20 August 2017, at:
fíle:///c:/users/user/desktop/
dii%20important/trabalhos%20dii%20importante/d
ii%20sexualidade%202016.pdf.

Bastos, F. S. (2013). *The person with a chronic illness: an explanatory theory on the problem of managing the illness and the therapeutic regime.* PhD Thesis, Portuguese Catholic University, Porto. Accessed on 11 August 2017 at:
http://repositorio.ucp.pt/bitstream/10400.14/11990/1/A%20pessoa%20com%20doen%C3%A7a%20cronica_Tese%20Doutoramento_Reitoria.pdf.

Burisch, J., Jess, T., Martinato, M. and Lakatos, P., L. (2013). The Burden of inflammatory bowel disease in Europe. *Journal of Crohn's and Colitis, 7, 322* 337.

Campolina, A. G., Dini, P. S. and Ciconeli, R. M. (2011). Impact of chronic disease on the quality of life of community-dwelling elderly in São Paulo (SP, Brazil). *Ciência e saúde coletiva*, 16 (6), 2919-2925. Accessed on September 20, 2017 at: http://www.scielo.br/pdf/csc/v16n6/29.pdf.

Campos, M. O. and Neto, J.F.R. (2008). Quality of life: an instrument for health promotion. *Revista Baiana de Saúde pública*, 32 (2), 232- 240.

Canavarro, M. C. and Vaz Serra, A. (2010). *Quality of life and health: an approach from the perspective of the World Health Organisation.* Lisbon. Calouste

Gulbenkian Foundation Edition.

Canuto, M. A. O., Nogueira, L. T. and Araújo, T. M. E. (2016). Health-related quality of life of people after stroke. *Acta Paul Enferm*, 29(3), 245-252.

Casellas, F., Lopez-Vivancos, J., Casado, A. and Malagelada, J. R. (2002). Factors affecting health-related quality of life of patients with inflammatory bowel disease. *Qual Life Res. Apr.* (11), 775-781.

Castro, E. K., Ponciano, C. F. and Pinto, D. W. (2010). Self-efficacy and quality of life of young adults with chronic diseases. *Aletheia,* 31, 137-148. Accessed on August 20, 2017 at:http://pepsic.bvsalud.org/pdf/aletheia/n31/n31a12.pdf.

Coelho, I. D. (2010). *Quality of Life and Inflammatory Bowel Disease, evaluation of a group of patients at the inflammatory bowel disease clinic of the cova da beira hospital centre.* Integrated master's thesis in medicine. University of Beira Interior. Accessed on 12 July 2017 at: file:///C:/Users/user/Downloads/isabeldiascoelhopdf%20(9).pdf.

Cohen, D., Bin, C. M. and Fayh, A. P. T. (2010). Assessment of quality of life of patients with Inflammatory Bowel Disease Residing in Southern Brazil. *Arq. Gastroenterol,* 47, (3), 285-289.

International Committee of Medical Journal Editors (2007). Uniform requirements for manuscripts submitted to medical journals: Vancouver standard. *Portuguese Journal of General Practice*, 23: 778-798. Accessed on 02 October 2017 at: https://infoscopio.files.wordpress.com/2008/02/norma_vancouver.pdf.

Cosnes, J., Gower-Rousseau, C., Seksik, P. and Cortot, A. (2011). Epidemiology and natural history of inflammatory bowel diseases. *Gastroenterology,* 140, (6), 1785-1794. Accessed on November 27, 2017 at: http://www.gastrojournal.org/article/S0016-5085(11)00164-8/pdf.

Costa, S., Tavares, M., Trindade, E. and Dias, J.A. (2012). Quality of life in paediatric inflammatory bowel disease: validation of the IMPACT III© questionnaire for the Portuguese population. *Acta Pediatr. Por.* 43 (5), 198-201.

Dantas, R. A. S., Sawada, N. N. and Malerbo, M. B. (2003). Research on quality of life: a review of scientific production at public universities in the state of São Paulo. *Rev. Latino-am. Enfermagem*, 11(4), 532-538. Accessed on 28 September 2017, at: http://www.scielo.br/pdf/rlae/v11n4/v11n4a17.pdf.

Order no. 9767(2014). Official Gazette, 2 (144), 19356. Accessed on 14 November 2017 at: file:///C:/Users/user/Downloads/i021975.pdf.

Directorate-General for Health (2015). *National Health Plan: revision and extension to 2020.* Lisbon: DGS. Accessed on 10 September 2017, at DGS: http://pns.dgs.pt/files/2015/06/Plano-Nacional-de-Saúde-Revisao-e-Extensao-a-2020.pdf.pdf

Dur, M., Sadlonova, M., Haider, S., Binder, A., Stoffer, M., Coenen, M., Smolen, J.,

Dejaco, C., Willer, A. K., Fialka-Moser, V., Moser, G. and Stamm, T. A. (2014). Health determinung concepts important to people with Crohn's disease and their coverage by patient-reported outcomes of health and wellbeing. *Journal of Crohn's and Colitis.* 8, (1), 45-55.

Farrukh, A. and Mayberry, J. F. (2014). Inflammatory bowel disease in Hispanic communities: a concerted South American approach could identify the aetiology of Crohn's disease and ulcerative colitis. *Arq Gastroenterol; ARQGA/1739,* 51(3), 271-275.

Fortin, M. F. (1999). *The Research Process, from conception to realisation.* Loures: Lusociência.

Fortin, M. F., Côté, J. and Filion, F. (2009). *Fundamentals and stages of the research process,* Loures: Lusodidacta.

Fróes, B.S.R. (2012). Conventional treatment in inflammatory bowel disease. *Revista do Hospital Universitário Pedro Ernesto, UERJ,* 27-32.

Gonçalves, J. D. O. (2010). *Quality of life of cancer patients undergoing surgery, satisfaction with care and information received during hospitalisation.* Master's dissertation. Faculty of Economics - University of Coimbra.

Gimenes, G.F. (2013). Uses and meanings of quality of life in contemporary health discourses. *Trab. Educ. Saúde, Rio de Janeiro,* 11(2), 291-318. Accessed on 23 September 2017 at:

http://www.scielo.br/pdf/tes/v11n2/a03v11n2.pdf.

Inflammatory Bowel Disease Study Group (2017). GEDII puts Portugal at the forefront of IBD debate and research, p.3-6. Accessed on July 04, 2017 at: http://perspetivas.pt/wp-content/uploads/2017/02/03-04-05-06.pdf.

Juillerat, P., Pittet. V., Bulliard, J., Guessous, I., Antonino, A. T., Mottet, C., Felley, C., Vader, J. and Michetti, P (2008). Prevalence of Inflammatory Bowel Disease in the Canton of Vaud (Switzerland): A population-based cohort study. *Journal of Crohn's and Colitis ,*2, 131-141.

Laverack, G. (2008). *Health promotion - power and empowerment.* Loures: Lusodidacta.

Lérias, C., Portela, F. and Pereira, S.J.A. (2000). Osteoporosis in inflammatory bowel disease. *GE - Portuguese Journal of Gastroenterology,*7, 203-214.

Loftus, E. V (2004). Clinical Epidemiology of Inflammatory Bowel Disease: Incidence, Prevalence, and Environmental Influences. *Gastroenterology,* 126, 1504-1517.

Lopes, H. L. (2014). *Crohn's disease: a challenge for nursing professionals.* Obtaining the title of Specialist in Nursing Care Lines. Federal University of Santa Catarina. Accessed on 23 September 2017 at:

https://repositorio.ufsc.br/bitstream/handle/123456789/170582/humberto%20le

al%20lopes-dcnt-tcc.pdf?sequence=1&isallowed=y.

Machado, C. M. C. (2013). *The nurse's contribution to health promotion and education in the general emergency service*. Dissertation prepared at the Technical University of Lisbon, Faculty of Human Motricity. Accessed on 17 September 2017 at:
https://www.repository.utl.pt/bitstream/10400.5/6986/1/Disserta%C3%A7%C3%A3o.pdf.

Magalhães, J., Castro, F. D., Carvalho, P.B., Machado, J. F., Leite, S., Moreira, et al. (2015). Disability in Inflammatory Bowel Disease: Translation to Portuguese and Validation of the "Inflammatory Bowel Disease - Disability Score". *GE Port J Gastroenterol*, 22, 4-14.

Marcon, S.S., Radovanovic, C.A.T., Waidman, M.A.P., Oliveira, M.L.F. and Sales, C.A. (2005). Experience and reflection of a study with families facing a chronic health situation. *Texto Contexto Enferm, Florianópolis,* 14(Esp.),116- 124.

Marques, M.A. (2012). *Resilience in situations of chronic illness*. São José de Itaperuna University Centre. Article presented to the Board of Examiners of the Psychology Course at the Centro Universitário São José de Itaperuna as a final requirement for obtaining the title of Psychologist. Accessed on 12 August, 2017 at: http://www.fsj.edu.br/wp-content/uploads/2013/11/Resili%C3%AAncia-na-situa%C3%A7%C3%A3o-de-doen%C3%A7as-cr%C3%B4nicas.pdf.

Martins, L. M., França, A. P. D. and Kimura, M. (1996). Quality of life of people with chronic illness. *Rev Latino-am.enfermagem, Ribeirão Preto,* 4 (3) 5-18.

Matos, L. and Figueiredo, N. P. (2013). *Fundamental gastroenterology*. Lda-Lousã. ISBN: 978-972-757-908-2.

Minayo, M. C. S., Hartz, Z. M. A. and Buss, P. M. (2000). Quality of life and health: A necessary debate. *Ciência & Saúde Coletiva*, 5(1), 7-18, 2000.

Ministry of Health (2006). *Mission for Primary Health Care. Glossary for family health units*. Lisbon: Ministry of Health. Accessed on 23 September 2017 at: http://www2.acss.min- saude.pt/Portals/0/ Glossario_USF.pdf.

Ministry of Health (2011). Manual of good practice, nursing. Instituto da Droga e da Toxicodependência, I. P. Accessed on 23 September 2017 at: http://www.sicad.pt/BK/Intervencao/TratamentoMais/Documentos%20Partilha dos/enfermag.pdf.

Molodecky, N. A., Soon, I. S., Rabi, D. M., Ghali, W A., Ferris, M., Chernoff, G., Benchimol, E.I., Panaccione, R., Ghosh, S., Barkema, H. W. and Kaplan, G. G. (2012). Increasing incidence and prevalence of the inflammatory bowel diseases with time, based on systematic review. *Gastroenterology,* 142 (1), 46-54. Accessed on November 01, 2017 at: http://www.gastrojournal.org/article/S0016-5085(11)01378-3/pdf.

Molodecky, N. A. and Kaplan G. G. (2010). Environmental Risk Factors for Inflammatory Bowel Disease. *Gastroenterol Hepatol*, 6 (5), 339-346. Accessed September 10, 1017 at: https://www.ncbi.nlm.nih.gov/ pmc/articles/ PMC2886488/.

Mowat, C., Cole, A., Windsor, A., Ahmad, T., Ian Arnott, I., Driscoll, R., Mitton, S., Orchard, T., Rutter, M., Younge, L., Lees, C., Ho, g., Satsangi J. and Bloom, S. (2011). On behalf of the IBD Section of the British Society of Gastroenterology. Guidelines for the management of inflammatory bowel disease in adults. *Gut.*

Neubauer, K.ɪ Arlukiewicz, A. and Paradowski, L. (2009). Quality of Life in Inflammatory Bowel Disease. *Adv Clin Exp Med*, 18(1), 79-83.

Neves, M. M. A. M. C. (2012). The role of nurses in the multidisciplinary team in primary health care - Systematic literature review. *Revista de Enfermagem Referência III Série,* (8), 125-134.

Neves, S.L.R. (2015). *Crisis experience in inflammatory bowel disease: a phenomenological-existential study.* Master's dissertation for a Master's degree in Clinical Specialisation. University Institute of Psychological, Social and Life Sciences. Lisbon. Accessed on 01 February, 2016 at: http://repositorio.ispa.pt/bitstream/10400.12/3968/1/18274.pdf.

Noronha, D. D., Martins, A. M. E. B. L., Dias, D. S., Silveira, M. F., Paula, A. M. B. and Haikal, D. S. A. (2016). Health-related quality of life among adults and associated factors: a population-based study. *Ciência & Saúde Coletiva,* 21 (2), 463-474.

Nunes, T., Fiorino, G., Danese, S and Sans, M. (2011). Familial aggregation in inflammatory bowel disease: is it genes or environment? *World J Gastroenterol*, 17, (22), 2715-2722. Accessed November 27, 2017 at: https://www.ncbi.nlm.nih.gov/pmc/articles/PMC3123468/

Oliveira, C; Antunes, C; Santos, C; Marques, A. and Sousa, M. (2017). Nutrition support in Crohn's disease. Nutrition support in Crohn's disease. *Acta Portuguesa de Nutrição*, 10 (2017) 44-48. Portuguese Nutrition Association.

Onal, i. k., Yuksel, E., Bayrakceken, K., Demir, M. M., Karaca, E. E., Ibis, M., Alizadeh, N., Sargin, Z. G., Hondur, A. M. and Arhan, M. (2015). Measurement and clinical implications of choroidal thickness in patients with inflammatory bowel disease. Determination of choroidal thickness and its clinical implications in patients with inflammatory bowel disease. *Arq Bras Oftalmol*, 78(5), 278282.

Order of Nurses (2001). *Nursing Care Quality Standards. Conceptual framework; descriptive statements.* Accessed on September 17, 2017 at OE:http://www.ordemenfermeiros.pt/publicacoes/Documents/ divulgar%20%20 padro%20de%20qualidade%20dos%20cuidados.pdf.

Ordem dos Enfermeiros (2010a). *Serving the community and ensuring quality: nurses at the forefront of chronic illness care.* International Council of Nurses. Order of Nurses edition. Accessed on 11 August 2017 at OE: http://www.ordemenfermeiros.pt/publicacoes/ documents/ kit_die_2010.pdf.

Ordem dos Enfermeiros (2010b). The Challenge of Chronic Diseases. Order of Nurses - *Regional Section of the Azores.* For the quality of nursing. Accessed on 30 November 2017 at OE: http://www.ordemenfermeiros.pt/sites/acores/artigospublicadoimpressalocal/Paginas/ODesafiodasDoenen%C3%A7asCronicas.aspx.

Ordem dos Enfermeiros (2011a). Regulation of quality standards for specialised care in Community and Public Health Nursing. Accessed on July 07, 2017 at OE: http://www.ordemenfermeiros.pt/colegios/documents/pqceecomunitsaudepublica.pdf.

Ordem dos Enfermeiros (2011b). Health Education, an Ally for Changing Behaviours. Ordem dos enfermeiros - *regional section, autonomous region of the Azores.* Nurses and...Health Education. Accessed on 23 September 2017 at OE:http://www.ordemenfermeiros.pt/sites/acores/ artigospublicadoimpressaloca l/Paginas/ OsEnfermeiroseeduca%C3%A7 %C3%A3oparaaSaude. aspx.

Ordem dos Enfermeiros (2011c). Coletânea de Comunicações Encontros, Simpósios, Painéis- *Secção Regional do Centro da Ordem dos Enfermeiros,* ISBN:978-989-97291-0-0. Accessed on 17 September 2017 at: http: www.ordemenfermeiros.pt/sites/centro/Documents/Colectanea%202008_2011. pdf.

Order of Nurses (2011d). Regulation no. 122 - Regulation of the Common Competences of the Specialist Nurse. *Diário da República, 2 (35), p. 8648-8653.* Accessed on 12 October 2017 at OE: http://www.aper.pt/Ficheiros/competencias%20comuns.pdf.

Order of Nurses (2011e). Regulation no. 128. Regulation of the Specific Competences of the Nurse Specialising in Community and Public Health Nursing. *Official Gazette, 2 (35), p.8667-8669.* Accessed on 18 September 2017 at OE: http://www.ordemenfermeiros.pt/faqs/Documents/Legislacao/Regulamento_128_2011.pdf.

World Health Organisation (2008). Primary health care: now more than ever: *World Health Report 2008.* Accessed on 21 September 2017 at: http://www.who.int/whr/2008/whr08_pr.pdf.

Palmela, C., Torres, J. and Cravo, M. (2015). New Trends in Inflammatory Bowel Disease. *GE. Port.J.Gastroenterol,* 22(3), 103-111.

Pereira, P., M., C. (2014). *Tobacco and inflammatory bowel disease.* Integrated master's thesis in medicine. Faculty of Medicine, University of Porto. Accessed

on 15 September 2017 at:
file:///C:/Users/user/Desktop/master/DII%20e%20o%20TABACO%202014.
pdf.

Pinto, C. and Ribeiro, J. L. P. (2006). The quality of life of cancer survivors. *Portuguese Journal of Public Health*, 24 (1), 37-56.

Pires, M. J. (2009). *Coronary heart disease risk factors and quality of life. An exploratory study in the municipality of Odivelas*. Master's dissertation in Health Communication. Universidade Aberta. Lisbon. Accessed on October 02, 2017 at:https://repositorioaberto.uab.pt/bitstream/10400.2/1432/1/Tese%20pdf%20 final.pdf.

Ponder, A. and Long, M.D. (2013). A clinical review of recent findings in the epidemiology of inflammatory bowel disease. *Clinicai Epidemiology, 5, 237* 247.

Pontes, R. M. A., Miszputen, S. J., Ferreira, O. F., Miranda, C. and Ferraz, M. B. (2004). Quality of life in patients with inflammatory bowel disease: translation into Portuguese and validation of the Inflammatory Bowel Disease Questionnaire (IBDQ). *Arq.Gastroenterol*, 41(2), 137-143.

Praça, M. I. F. (2012). *Health-related quality of life: the perspective of users attending the Health Centres of the ACES Trás-os-Montes I Nordeste*. Master's dissertation. Associação de Politécnicos do Norte - Instituto Politécnico de Bragança, Bragança.

Quina, M. G, and Collaborators (2000). *Clinical gastroenterology*. Lousã: Lidel.

Ramos, A., Calvet, X., Sicilia, B., Vergara, M., Figuerola, A., Motos, J., Sastre, A., Villoria, A. and Gomollo, F. (2015). IBD-related work disability in the community: Prevalence, severity and predictive factors. A cross-sectional study. *United European Gastroenterology Journal*, 3 (4), 335-342.

Raposo, F. A. Q. (2008). *Inflammatory bowel disease*. Master's thesis submitted to the Faculty of Health Sciences, University of Beira Interior, Covilhã. Accessed on August, 20, 2017 at:
file:///C:/Users/user/Downloads/filiparaposo_mestrad%20(8).pdf.

National Hospital Speciality and Referral Network (2016). *Gastroenterology and Hepatology*. Accessed on 27 August 2017 at: https://www.sns.gov.pt/wp-content/uploads/2016/11/RRH- Gasteroenterologia_hepatologia.pdf.

Russell, M. (2000). Changes in the incidence of inflammatory bowel disease: What does it mean? *European Journal of Internal Medicine,* 11 (4), 191-196.

Sampaio, A. C. L. (2007). *Benefits of walking on the quality of life of adults*. Degree dissertation presented at the Faculty of Sport of the University of Porto.

Santos, A. A. L., Dorna, S. M., Vulcano, B. S. D., Augusti, L., Franzoni, C.L., Gondo, F.F., Romeiro, F.G. and Sassaki, L. Y. (2015). *Nutritional* therapy in inflammatory bowel diseases: *Review article Nutrire*, 40 (3), 383-396. Accessed on 22 October 2017 at: http://sban.cloudpainel.com.br/ files/ revistas_publicacoes/486.pdf.

Santos, G. M., Silva, L. R. and Santana, G. O. (2014). Nutritional repercussions in children and adolescents in the presence of inflammatory bowel diseases. *Rev Paul Pediatr, 32* (4), 403-411. Accessed on 17 September 2017 at: http://www.scielo.br/pdf/rpp/v32n4/pt_0103-0582-rpp-32-04-00403.pdf.

Santos, M. F. C. (2015). *Sleep disturbance in children with inflammatory bowel disease. Is there a relationship?* Integrated Master's Degree in Medicine, Faculty of Medicine, University of Lisbon. Accessed on 19 October 2017 at: http://repositorio.ul.pt/jspui/bitstream/10451/25798/1/MafaldaFCSantos.pdf.

Santos, S., Santos, E., Ferrão, A. and Figueiredo, C. (2011). The impact of chronic illness on adolescence. *Nascer e Crescer*, 20 (1), 16-19. Accessed on October 02, 2017 at: http://www.scielo.mec.pt/pdf/nas/v20n1/v20n1a03.pdf.

Sarlo, R. S., Barreto, C. R. and Domingues, T. A. M. (2008). Understanding the experience of patients with Crohn's disease. *Acta Paul Enferm* 2008, 21 (4), 62935.

Saurabh, K and Ahuja, V. (2017). Epidemiology of Inflammatory Bowel Disease in India: The Great Shift East . *Inflamm Intest Dis,* pp.1-14. DOI: 10.1159/000465522.

Silva, A. F., Schieferdecker, M. E. M. and Amarante, H. M. B. S. (2011). Dietary intake in patients with inflammatory bowel disease. *ABCD Arq Bras cir dig*, 24(3), 204-209.

Silva, I., C., L. (2015). *Health-related quality of life in patients with inflammatory bowel disease treated with biological therapy.* Dissertation submitted to the Faculty of Medicine, Universidade Estadual Paulista "Júlio de Mesquita Filho", Câmpus de Botucatu. Accessed on July 14, 2017 at: https://repositorio.unesp.br/bitstream/handle/11449/128144/000849094.pdf?sequence=1

Simão, P. L (2014). *Therapeutic Guidelines for the Treatment of Crohn's Disease* Dissertation in Pharmaceutical Sciences. University of Algarve Faculty of Science and Technology. Accessed on 24 August 2017 at: https://sapientia.ualg.pt/bitstream/10400.1/8139/1/Disserta%C3%A7%C3%A3 the_Master_Philippe_Sim%C3%A3o.pdf

Smeltzer, C. S., Bare, G. B., Hinkle, L. J. and Cheever, H. K. (2011). *Bruner & Suddarth. Treatise on Medical-Surgical Nursing.* 12 (1) Rio de Janeiro: Editora, Guanabara, Koogan LTDA.

Sousa, M. R. M. G. C., Martins, T. and Pereira, F. (2015). O refletir das práticas dos enfermeiros na abordagem à pessoa com doença crónica. *Revista de*

Enfermagem Referência Série IV, (6), 55-63.

Souza, M. S., Barbosa, D. A., Espinosa, M. M. and Belasco, A. G. S. (2011). Quality of life of patients with inflammatory bowel disease. *Acta Paul Enferm ;24 (4), 479-484.*

Souza, M. M., Belasco, A. G. S. and Aguilar-nascimento, J. E. (2008). Epidemiological Profile of Patients with Inflammatory Bowel Disease in the State of Mato Grosso. *Rev Bras Coloproct,* 28 (3), 324-328.

Stanhope, M. and Lancaster, J. (2010). *Public Health Nursing: Population-Centred Health Care in the Community* (7ª ed.). Loures: Lusociência.

Torres, J. A. P., Santana; R. M., Torres, F. A. P., Moura, A. R. and Neto, J. R. T. (2011). Inflammatory bowel diseases at the University Hospital of the Federal University of Sergipe: extraintestinal manifestations. *Rev bras Coloproct*, 31, (2), 115-119.

Trindade, I. A., Ferreira, C. and Gouveia, J. P. (2016). Inflammatory bowel disease: The harmful mechanism of experiential avoidance for patients' quality of life. *Journal of health Psychology,* 21 (12), 2882-2892.

Valério, F., Cutait, R., Sipahi, A., Damião, A. and Leite, K. (2006). Cancer in Crohn's Disease: Case Report. *Rev bras Coloproct*, 26 (4), 443-446.

Verissimo, R. (2008). *Quality of Life in Inflammatory Bowel Disease*: Psychometric Evaluation of an IBDQ Cross-Culturally Adapted Version. *J Gastrointestin Liver Dis*, 17 (4), 439-444.

Vintém, J. M. (2008). National Health Surveys: self-perception of health status: a gender and schooling analysis. *Portuguese Journal of Public Health,* 26 (2), 5-15.

Watson, J. (2002). *Nursing: human science and caring. A theory of nursing.* Loures: Lusociência.

World Gastroenterology Organisation Practice Guidelines (2015). *Inflammatory bowel disease*. WGO Practice Guidelines IBD. Accessed on September 02, 2017 at: http://www.worldgastroenterology.org/ UserFiles/file/ guidelines/ inflammatory- bowel-disease-portuguese-2015.pdf.

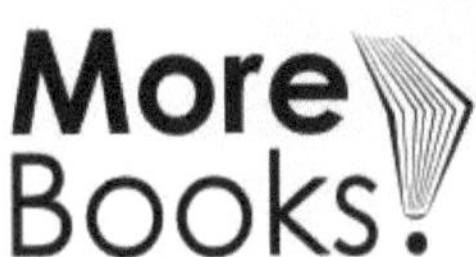

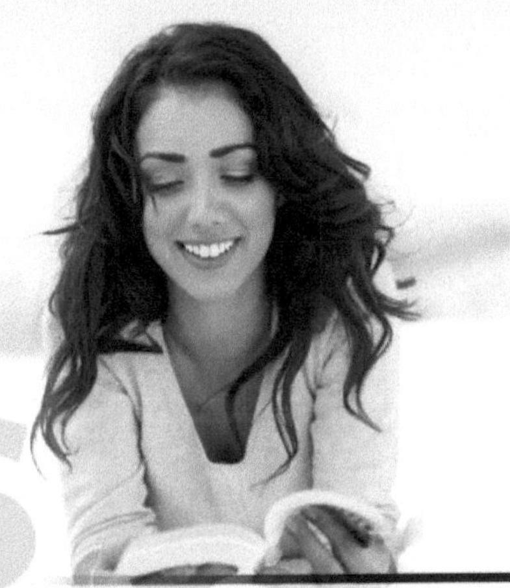

I want morebooks!

Buy your books fast and straightforward online - at one of world's fastest growing online book stores! Environmentally sound due to Print-on-Demand technologies.

Buy your books online at
www.morebooks.shop

Kaufen Sie Ihre Bücher schnell und unkompliziert online – auf einer der am schnellsten wachsenden Buchhandelsplattformen weltweit! Dank Print-On-Demand umwelt- und ressourcenschonend produzi ert.

Bücher schneller online kaufen
www.morebooks.shop

info@omniscriptum.com
www.omniscriptum.com

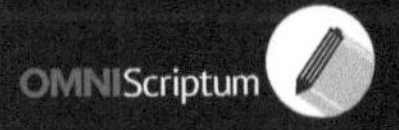

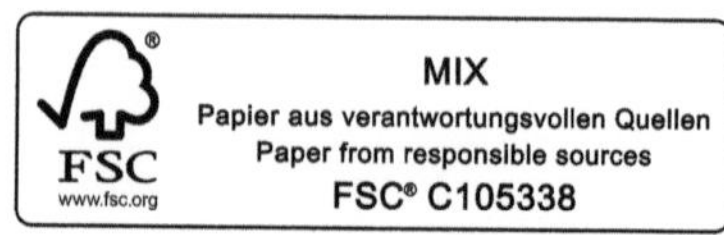
FSC
www.fsc.org
MIX
Papier aus verantwortungsvollen Quellen
Paper from responsible sources
FSC® C105338